The 7 Stages of Alzheimer's Disease

Walking Betty Home

Lessons from 11 Years as a Caregiver

Joshua T. Pettit

Forward by:
Charles "Bob" Pettit

Table of Contents

FOREWORD
By Charles "Bob" Pettit

*"Dementia does not only change
the one who forgets, it transforms
the one who stays."*

Dementia is a word many people fear, yet few truly understand it until it steps into their own lives. It arrives quietly in the early stages, disguised as forgetfulness or distraction. It creeps into daily routines, into conversations, into relationships, altering them not all at once, but in small, steady waves. And for those who walk alongside someone living with dementia, the journey becomes far more than a medical diagnosis. It becomes a lesson in love, in patience, in grief, in resilience, and in the sacredness of presence.

This book was written for every person who has ever loved someone through dementia.

For the caregivers who rise each morning with courage.

For the families who navigate change with trembling hands.

For the sons and daughters who become protectors.

For the spouses who remain constant companions.

For anyone who has ever held the hand of someone forgetting but still deserving of compassion and dignity.

Dementia is not simply a clinical condition; it is a lived experience. It affects not only the one diagnosed, but everyone who loves them. The emotional weight of this journey is heavy, and too often caregivers carry it in silence. This book seeks to break that silence. It seeks to name the stages, to explain the science in plain and accessible language, but also to honor the humanity behind every symptom and every struggle.

You will not find judgment in these pages.

You will not find cold medical jargon or impersonal advice.

Instead, you will find stories; real, tender, heartbreaking, and beautiful. You will find clarity where confusion once lived. You will find guidance where fear once stood. You will find comfort in the knowledge that you are not alone.

Every stage of dementia reveals something about the human spirit: its fragility, yes, but also its strength. Its vulnerability, but also its capacity for connection.

Its decline, but also the enduring presence of love.

If you are walking this path right now, let this book be a companion. Let it sit with you in the hard moments. Let it remind you that your emotions are valid, your exhaustion is understandable, and your love is extraordinary.

If dementia has already taken someone you loved, may these pages bring healing. May they help you make sense of what you witnessed. May they validate your grief and honor your devotion.

And if you simply wish to understand dementia better, may this book open your heart to those who live with it every day, and to the caregivers who quietly shoulder some of the heaviest burdens on earth.

Dementia changes people, yes, but it also changes those who love them. And sometimes, the greatest transformation happens not in the person with the disease, but in the one who stays.

This book is a testament to that kind of love.

The kind that endures decline.

The kind that survives forgetting.

The kind that grows deeper even as memories fade.

The kind that holds on, with tenderness, until the very end.

May this journey through the seven stages bring you wisdom, strength, compassion, and above all, peace.

ABOUT THE AUTHOR:
JOSHUA PETTIT

*"I did not set out to become an advocate,
I simply loved my mother... and stayed."*

Joshua Pettit never set out to become a caregiver, an advocate, or the voice behind one of the most recognized Alzheimer's caregiving journeys on social media. He was simply a devoted son, one who loved his mother, Betty, and father, Bob, fiercely and without condition. When Alzheimer's disease entered their lives, it reshaped everything, and Josh stepped into a role that would not only define the next decade of his life but also touch millions of hearts around the world.

For 11 years, Josh and his father cared for Betty, walking with her through every stage of Alzheimer's. The last years of her life were spent in Josh's home, where he, along with his father, Bob, became her full-time caregiver, providing her a home, cooking her meals, helping her bathe and dress, soothing her fears, redirecting her confusion, and comforting her during the long, difficult nights that dementia so often brings. He was not perfect; he would tell you, but he was present. He showed up. Again, and again. And that was enough.

In 2022, one simple, tender moment changed everything.

Betty stood before a full-length mirror, speaking to her reflection as if she were greeting an old friend. Josh recorded the moment, not for fame, but to document the beauty and heartbreak of dementia.

When he shared the video on TikTok, something extraordinary happened. The world fell in love with Betty. Her innocence, humor, tenderness, and vulnerability resonated with millions. The clip went viral, and the Pettit family's life changed overnight.

Suddenly, Josh found himself with a rapidly growing audience, 1.3 million followers and counting, people who didn't just watch but also connected deeply with Betty and her journey.

Through his posts, Josh offered something rare: **real caregiving, unfiltered and full of love**. He shared their daily routines, the small victories, the painful declines, and most importantly, the profound humanity that still lived within Betty despite her illness.

News outlets and journalists began to take notice. Josh and Betty's story appeared on CNN, People Magazine, Business Insider, The Daily Mail, The Charlotte Observer, Local Television News, and beyond. They became symbols of what caregiving truly looks like, the frustration, the grace, the humor, the heartbreak, and the unwavering devotion.

But the fame was never the point.

The point was connection.

The point was education.

The point was love.

When Betty died at the age of 86, thousands around the world mourned with Josh and his father. Her passing marked the end of an extraordinary caregiving chapter, but it also marked the beginning of a new mission for Josh: **sharing everything he had learned so that other families would feel less alone.**

After her death, Josh and his father turned their grief into legacy. Together they co-wrote three books:

- ***I'm Betty: A Woman's Battle with Alzheimer's Disease, Rise to Social Media Fame, and Her Family's Caregiving Journey*** — a heartfelt memoir of Betty's life, their family's caregiving experience, and the unexpected global impact of her story.

- ***He's My Guy: Bob's Story*** — an intimate look at his father's life, resilience, and role as both husband and caregiver.

- ***The Adventures of Miss Betty's Flat Teddy*** — a children's book which teaches about Alzheimer's disease and outlines the adventures of a Flat Teddy that was sent to Betty as a gift

These books were not written for sympathy or attention, they were written to honor Betty, to support other families, and to remind the world that behind every diagnosis is a person with dignity and a family doing the best they can.

A portion of the proceeds from every book sold was donated to the Alzheimer's Association. As of this writing, they have raised **over $100,000** for the Alzheimer's Association in Betty's honor.

Now, with this book on understanding dementia and caregiving, Josh continues his mission. He brings not only research and explanation; but lived experience, long nights, tearful moments, tender memories, raw honesty, and the kind of wisdom only earned through years of caregiving.

He writes so that:
caregivers feel seen,
families feel supported,
loved ones feel understood, and
no one has to navigate dementia alone.

Josh's voice is not that of a distant expert but of a fellow traveler, someone who has walked the path, stumbled on it, cried on it, and learned to keep going anyway. His insight is shaped by experience, yes, but far more by love.

Today, Josh continues to advocate for Alzheimer's awareness, caregiver support, and compassionate education. He speaks from experience, from heartache, and from a place of deep empathy. His work honors Betty's legacy and stands as a testament to the enduring bond between parent and child.

To millions, Josh is a storyteller.

To caregivers, he is a companion.

To families in crisis, he is reassurance.

To the memory of his mother, he is love in action.

But at his core, Joshua Pettit is simply a son, a son who walked his mother home with courage, tenderness, and grace.

And through his writing, he now walks with you, too.

STAGE 1:
THE SILENT BEGINNING

*"The beginning of dementia is not
something you witness in real time,
it is something you recognize only after
everything has changed, when you look back
and realize the silence had already begun."*

Most stories begin with a clear starting point, a first line, the opening scene, the moment something changes. Dementia is not that kind of story. If anything, dementia begins like a whisper in another room, too soft to hear, too faint to notice, too far away to understand.

Stage One, known formally as **No Impairment**, is the stage before the world shifts. It is the final chapter of "before," even though no one knows they are living inside it.

If you've ever walked back through your memories, retracing steps to figure out when dementia truly started, this is the stage you were searching for. But Stage One leaves no breadcrumbs. No trail. No clues. It is a quiet beginning inside the brain, a slow rearranging of microscopic details that no ordinary person could see or feel.

The Illusion of Normalcy

During Stage One, life looks perfectly ordinary. The person wakes up, drinks their coffee, checks their calendar, completes their chores, carries conversations, remembers birthdays, pays bills, runs errands, gets annoyed by traffic, watches their favorite shows, and tells their familiar jokes. Nothing about them appears changed, strained, or lost.

They are fully themselves.

Friends see them the same way. Family sees them the same way. Doctors see nothing wrong. Even advanced memory testing shows no signs of cognitive decline.

Stage One feels like a still lake, calm, reflective, undisturbed, giving no hint that something is about to ripple across its surface.

But the brain is a complex landscape, and disturbances often begin long before the water breaks.

What's Happening Beneath the Surface

To understand Stage One, imagine the brain as one of the busiest cities in the world; millions of roads (neural pathways), billions of vehicles (electrical signals), and countless intersections controlling the flow of information.

Every thought, memory, movement, emotion, and decision depends on these roads functioning smoothly.

Now imagine that in one tiny neighborhood of that city, a construction project begins without anyone noticing. A few sidewalks crack. A section of pavement weakens. Traffic still moves as it normally would, so the city doesn't feel any different. But the foundation is shifting in ways no outsider can see.

This is what happens in Stage One.

Protein Changes Begin Quietly

Most forms of dementia, especially Alzheimer's disease, begin with the silent buildup of two problematic proteins:

- **Beta-amyloid** (forms sticky plaques between neurons)
- **Tau protein** (forms twisted tangles inside neurons)

In a healthy brain, amyloid and tau serve important functions. They support cellular structure, communication, and repair. But when they misfold, they create debris, like trash left on the roads and inside the buildings of our metaphorical city.

In Stage One:
- Plaques begin collecting between neurons
- Tangles begin forming inside neurons
- Synapses (the tiny spaces between neurons) begin to weaken
- Communication becomes slightly less efficient
- The brain quietly adapts and rewires itself to compensate

None of this creates symptoms yet. The brain is extraordinarily resilient. It works overtime to hide these early changes.

The person living in Stage One feels completely normal because the brain makes life feel normal.

How Early Changes Hide Themselves
The human brain is a master of disguise.

When one neural pathway becomes weak, the brain uses another. When a neuron dies, surrounding neurons pick up the slack. When communication slows, the brain temporarily boosts chemical messengers to maintain function.

This ability is called **neuroplasticity**: the power of the brain to adapt, repair, reroute, and reorganize.

In Stage One, neuroplasticity does all the heavy lifting. It keeps the symptoms buried, the exterior unchanged, and the illusion of normalcy fully intact.

To the world, and to the person themselves, everything feels right.

Why Stage One Can Last for Years

Many scientists believe Stage One can last 20 years or more before symptoms appear. Dementia is not a fast-moving storm. It is a slow, steady change that begins decades before it is ever recognized.

Consider these facts:

- Amyloid plaques begin forming **10–20 years before** symptoms
- Tau tangles begin forming **10–15 years before** symptoms
- Brain shrinkage (atrophy) often starts **long before** diagnosis
- Blood vessels in the brain **may already be** weakening
- Inflammation may be quietly **increasing**

But because the brain compensates so well, the person remains fully themselves: capable, sharp, independent.

If you are caring for someone with dementia now, it is almost certain that Stage One happened long before you noticed anything. And that is **not your fault**. That is simply the nature of the disease.

When Caregivers Look Back
One of the most painful parts of dementia caregiving is the reflection—the mental reviewing of moments, behaviors, conversations, or "odd little things" from years past.

We ask ourselves:
- "Was that the beginning?"
- "Should I have noticed something sooner?"
- "Was that missed appointment the first sign?"
- "Was that moment of forgetfulness something more?"

But Stage One whispers defiantly: There was nothing to notice. You could not have known.

This is one of the most important messages caregivers must hear. **Dementia is not something you catch early because you were especially observant.** It's something that remains hidden until the brain cannot hide it anymore.

Stage One absolves caregivers from years of guilt they never deserved.

The Biology of a Silent Stage

Let's explore the medical side a bit deeper, still in simple terms, because understanding the "why" gives a sense of grounding.

1. Neurons Begin to Change

Neurons are the brain's messengers, sending electrical signals to communicate. In Stage One:

- Some neurons begin to misfire
- Some lose shape
- Some develop mild structural instability

But the changes are so small that the surrounding networks compensate.

2. Synapses Become Less Efficient

Synapses are the communication points between neurons. Early dementia causes:

- Slower signal transmission
- Slightly weaker connections
- Decreased neurotransmitters (like acetylcholine)

Still, nothing is strong enough to cause visible symptoms.

3. Inflammation Increases

The brain's immune cells, called microglia, activate more often during early dementia. They try to "clean up" plaques and tangles. Over time, this constant activation creates inflammation.

In Stage One, inflammation is mild, but it marks the beginning of a long-term struggle inside the brain.

4. Blood Flow Subtly Changes

Blood vessels may slightly stiffen or narrow. The brain receives slightly less blood, but again, not enough for anyone to notice.

The person still remembers.

Still thinks.

Still functions.

Still lives fully.

Because the brain is fighting hard behind the scenes to stay afloat.

The Person in Stage One

It's important to remember that Stage One is not dementia as we think of it. It is not memory loss, confusion, wandering, or caregiving. It is not forgetting your own children or misplacing your keys three times a day.

In Stage One:
- The person is perfectly normal
- The brain is compensating
- The disease is present, but invisible
- Life feels unchanged

This is the last stage where the world remains whole, familiar, and unbroken.

How Families Experience Stage One

Families never recognize Stage One as part of dementia. They simply experience these years as "normal years."

It is only later, sometimes much later, that caregivers look back with heartache and wonder if something was already unraveling in the background.

Stage One allows life to go on untouched. That is its blessing and its burden.

If We Could See Stage One

If we had a window into the brain during Stage One, we would see:
- A storm forming far offshore
- A slow accumulation of clouds on the horizon
- Subtle shifts in pressure

But from the shore, from the outside, the sky still looks blue.

Dementia begins quietly so people can continue living life without fear. This stage is a mercy, even if it is misunderstood.

The Dignity of the Unseen
There is dignity in Stage One.

The person still:
- Dreams
- Loves
- Works
- Laughs
- Learns
- Belongs
- Leads
- Creates

They are unburdened by the knowledge of what is happening inside their brain.

Their story is still their own, unshared with disease.

Why Understanding Stage One Matters
Most families only enter the story at Stage Three or Four, when symptoms finally appear. They never see Stage One or Two. They don't know what was happening silently for years.

Understanding Stage One helps caregivers:

- Release misplaced guilt
- Appreciate that **dementia is not sudden**
- Understand the biological timeline
- Realize they did nothing wrong
- Recognize how long the brain fought before symptoms appeared

Stage One is the brain's quiet resilience before it begins to falter.

The End of Stage One

There is no visible end to Stage One. The transition into Stage Two is seamless, unnoticeable, and without warning.

If you're looking for a dramatic moment where the story "begins," dementia will not give you one.

It begins invisibly.

Moves quietly.

Hides skillfully.

Until one day, the whispers grow louder, and a family begins to sense that something has shifted. That is Stage Two.

STAGE 2:
THE WHISPERS OF CHANGE

*"The earliest signs of dementia rarely
feel frightening. They feel ordinary,
explainable, almost harmless,
which is why they are so easy to dismiss,
and so painful to recognize later."*

Stage Two is the first place where the earliest hints of dementia surface, not loudly, not clearly, but softly. This is the stage where memory begins to slip in ways that feel just a little "off," but nothing alarming. It is the beginning of doubt, not diagnosis. Families do not see this stage as dementia; they see it as a person getting older, being distracted, overwhelmed, or tired.

If Stage One was the silent beginning, Stage Two is the soft tap on the shoulder: the stage where the disease begins to murmur, not yet confident enough to identify itself, but bold enough to make its presence known in tiny, forgettable ways.

Every caregiver I've ever met eventually looks back at Stage Two with clarity they didn't have at the time. They say, "Oh... I think this is when it really started."

But recognizing Stage Two while you're in it? **Nearly impossible.**

Let's step into this stage, slowly and gently, and explore what begins to shift in both the brain and the person living with dementia.

The Subtle Changes of Stage Two
In Stage Two, also called **Very Mild Cognitive Decline**, the symptoms are barely noticeable. They are not strong enough to disrupt daily life or to raise red flags. But they are persistent enough, in hindsight, to mark the earliest on-the-surface signs that something deeper is beginning to change within the brain.

These changes include:
- Misplacing items a little more often
- Taking slightly longer to recall names
- Forgetting which word you were about to say
- Needing to retrace steps
- Losing your train of thought more frequently
- Feeling "foggy" or "scattered" at times

Every single one of these changes can be explained by normal aging…

Which is why Stage Two is almost always ignored.

The truth is simple, at this stage, **you cannot tell if the symptoms are dementia or just the natural wear-and-tear of a human brain** that has lived many busy years.

Even doctors consider Stage Two ambiguous.

The Brain in Stage Two: Changes We Can't See
To understand Stage Two, we first need to zoom in, deep inside the brain, to witness the earliest outward consequences of the silent processes that began in Stage One.

1. Synaptic Efficiency Begins to Decline
Synapses are the tiny gaps where signals pass from one neuron to another. In early dementia:
- Signals move more slowly
- Fewer connections fire at once
- Some connections don't fire at all

This doesn't stop the person from functioning normally; it just means some memories take a bit longer to surface.

Think of a computer with too many tabs open.

It still works, but it might lag a little.

2. Short-Term Memory Begins to Show Strain
In Stage Two, the first area commonly affected is the hippocampus, the brain's memory center.

It becomes just slightly less efficient at:
- Forming new memories
- Organizing information
- Retrieving recently stored facts

The person doesn't forget major life events. They forget:

- Where they set their glasses
- Why they walked into a room
- What they did yesterday afternoon

Still subtle, still explainable, still easy to dismiss.

3. Neuroplasticity Still Compensates... For Now
Just like in Stage One, the brain compensates beautifully. When one pathway weakens, the brain reroutes through another, like a driver avoiding a small crack in the road by shifting lanes.

But compensation has limits, and Stage Two is the first stage where these limits begin to thin, just enough for micro-symptoms to slip through.

4. Amyloid Plaques and Tau Tangles Increase
A healthy brain continuously clears out proteins, waste, and damaged cells. But in dementia, the cleanup process loses ground.

More amyloid plaques begin sticking between neurons.

More tau tangles form inside neurons.

Still, symptoms remain subtle. But these build-ups are like termites in a house, you don't see the damage until much later, even though the weakening has already begun.

What the Person Experiences
By Stage Two, most people feel that something is slightly different, but they don't see it as a medical problem.

Common thoughts include:
- "I'm just tired."
- "I've been so busy lately."
- "Must be stress."
- "I guess this is what getting older feels like."
- "My mind is just full today."

Remember: these people are not losing important memories yet.

They're losing the edges, little pieces of information that don't feel essential.

Subtle But Significant
A person in Stage Two still:
- Holds conversations normally
- Drives safely
- Manages finances
- Cooks meals
- Works jobs

- Maintains hobbies
- Uses technology

They are fully independent.

But they occasionally feel like their brain is "working harder" than it used to. They may hesitate before answering questions. They may pause to recollect a detail that once would have been immediate.

This hesitation is Stage Two's calling card.

What Loved Ones Experience
Almost nothing.

Stage Two is extremely easy to miss because the symptoms resemble natural forgetfulness. Families simply don't notice anything pathological.

If you think back on your loved one, you might remember:
- More repetitive questions
- A few forgotten appointments
- More misplaced objects
- Increased reliance on reminders
- Moments where they seemed "distracted"
- Times they struggled to find a word

But in the moment, these didn't seem alarming. They seemed normal.

And that is exactly why Stage Two is known as one of dementia's "invisible stages."

A Story From This Stage

My mother, Betty, had always been sharp. Sharp as a tack. She ran a household like a well-oiled machine: balancing schedules, managing finances, planning meals, and keeping everyone in line in a way that only she could. She was deeply involved in her church, active in countless nonprofit groups, and the force that quietly held our family together.

She remembered birthdays without writing them down.

She kept mental lists of everyone's favorite foods.

She could recite recipes from her childhood without ever opening a cookbook.

She was quick-witted, social, funny, and wonderfully organized.

That was the woman we knew. The woman we trusted. The woman whose memory seemed unshakable.

During her early retirement, she and my father set off to live their dream, traveling full-time in an RV, seeing the country, meeting new people, and enjoying the freedom they had earned. With this new chapter came new details: a North Carolina cell phone number, my home address for mail, a life that no longer relied on the same familiar information she had used for thirty years.

And that's when we first noticed it.

If someone asked for her phone number, she hesitated.

If someone asked for her address, she'd glance at Dad.

When required to give her Social Security number or her mother's maiden name, she sometimes mixed them up, occasionally giving her own maiden name instead.

She laughed it off every time. So did we.

"It's new information."

"It's not something I use often."

"Your father takes care of all that."

And honestly? It sounded reasonable.

After all, who remembers a new phone number right away? Who recites an address they rarely use? And who among us hasn't had a "senior moment" here and there?

We teased her the way families do.

We shrugged it off as **normal aging**.

We reassured ourselves that she was still sharp in every other area, and she truly was.

She cooked like a master.

She socialized effortlessly.

She told stories with detail and humor.

She navigated the RV lifestyle with no trouble at all.

From the outside, nothing looked concerning.

But now, looking back, we see it clearly. Betty couldn't hold onto new information anymore. Her brain wasn't filing it the way it used to.

Old memories stayed strong.

New ones slipped through her fingers.

We didn't know it then, but these were the first tiny cracks in the foundation. The earliest signs that something subtle, but significant, was beginning to change.

At the time, it didn't alarm us.

It didn't disrupt her life.

It didn't take anything valuable away.

It just... *whispered*.

And we couldn't yet hear what it was saying.

Betty didn't know it yet, but she was standing at the threshold of dementia.

Not inside it.

Not swallowed by it.

Just standing on the doorstep, hand on the knob, unaware that the door was quietly beginning to open.

That is Stage Two.

Stage Two is one of the most deceptive stages of dementia, because everything still feels normal. The person you love still looks like themselves, acts like themselves, and functions like themselves. The changes are so small, so inconsistent, so easily explained away, that no one thinks to worry.

In Stage Two, dementia doesn't take anything obvious.

It doesn't erase abilities.

It doesn't disrupt daily life.

It simply begins loosening the threads, one subtle slip at a time.

Losing a new phone number isn't alarming.

Mixing up addresses seems harmless.

Forgetting seldom-used details feels normal.

Because dementia at this stage hides behind logic.

Behind humor.

Behind "Oh, I just forgot."

It allows the person you love to continue living fully, while quietly rearranging the wiring in the background. It is not painful. It is not frightening. It is not even recognizable.

But it is the beginning.

When I think back on Mom laughing off those forgotten details, I realize now that her confidence hadn't changed, just her ability to store new information. She relied on old memories because she trusted them. She avoided new ones because they slipped away before she could hold onto them.

And we, loving her, admiring her, believing in her, missed the signs entirely.

Not because we weren't paying attention.

But because **Stage Two is designed to be missed**.

It is the softest part of the journey.

The quietest.

The most innocent.

A stage where life still feels whole, even as subtle changes begin to whisper that something deeper is starting.

Stage Two is the doorway.

And while none of us recognized it at the time, this was where Mom first stepped onto the path; gentle, unnoticed, and already moving toward a future we were not yet ready to imagine.

Why Stage Two Is So Hard to Identify
The human brain changes naturally with age. Scientists call this "normal cognitive aging," and it includes:
- Slightly slower processing
- Occasional forgetfulness
- Decreased multitasking abilities
- Reduced mental "sharpness" during fatigue

Because these changes are expected, Stage Two hides behind them.

Even professionals struggle to distinguish Normal aging from Very early dementia.

It's simply too subtle.

A neurologist can only diagnose dementia at this stage with highly detailed cognitive testing or advanced imaging, and even then, nothing is 100% certain.

Most diagnoses don't begin until Stage Three or Four.

The Person's Inner World During Stage Two
People in Stage Two often begin to sense:
- Moments of uncertainty
- A slight uneasiness about memory
- A heightened awareness of simple mistakes
- Frustration at feeling "slower"

Emotionally, Stage Two may include:
- Mild embarrassment ("I used to remember everything.")
- Anxiety ("Why am I forgetting little things?")
- Denial ("I'm just tired.")
- Overcompensation ("Let me make more lists so I don't forget.")

No one in Stage Two thinks, "I'm getting dementia."

Not yet.

They think, "I'm slipping a little, but I'll be okay."

They still trust their mind.

They still trust their independence.

They still trust their memory, despite its occasional hiccups.

How Stage Two Affects Daily Life
Here's the truth: It doesn't.

Not in any meaningful or disruptive way.

People in Stage Two:
- Live alone safely
- Cook safely
- Drive safely
- Manage finances
- Keep their schedule
- Maintain relationships
- Enjoy hobbies

But... they start making small adjustments:

1. More Lists
Grocery lists, to-do lists, reminder notes.

Little safety nets.

2. More Rechecking
Making sure the stove is off twice.

Verifying appointments multiple times.

3. More Frustration
"You know that person... what's her name... from down the street..."

4. More Covering-Up
Laughing off forgetfulness.

Changing the subject when memory fails.

Using phrases like, "You know what I mean."

These are not signs of disability.

They are signs of strain, just a tiny bit, on a cognitive system that once operated effortlessly.

What Caregivers Should Know About This Stage
While Stage Two doesn't require caregiving, it requires awareness.

Not suspicion.

Not anxiety.

Not diagnosis-hunting.

Just awareness.

Here's what helps most:

1. Don't Jump to Conclusions
Forgetfulness is normal. Dementia-like symptoms do not automatically mean dementia.

2. Don't Call Out Every Mistake
People remember how you make them feel.

Being corrected constantly makes them feel incompetent.

3. Don't Use Scare Language

Avoid:

- "You're losing your mind."
- "You need to get checked."
- "You're getting forgetful."

Even if meant jokingly, these comments can plant fear.

4. Be Gently Observant

Not critical or suspicious, just aware.

5. Encourage Cognitive Health

Without alarming them, support brain-healthy activities:

- Social interaction
- Physical exercise
- Balanced diet
- Mental engagement
- Adequate sleep

6. Keep an Eye on Patterns

One forgotten appointment is no big deal.

Patterns are what matter.

7. But Above All: Show Grace

People in Stage Two are not "slipping away."

They are still here.

Still capable.

Still independent.

Still themselves.

They simply experience moments where their brain tugs a little slower than before.

The Transition Into Stage Three
Stage Two slowly bleeds into Stage Three.

There is no moment where you wake up and say, "We crossed into the next stage."

Instead, the changes become:
- More consistent
- More noticeable
- More difficult to explain away

Loved ones start saying:
- "You already told me that."
- "Didn't we talk about this yesterday?"
- "You forgot again?"

The person starts to feel the changes more deeply, more personally.

Stage Two is the whisper, but Stage Three is the first time that dementia truly clears its throat.

STAGE 3:
WHEN THE SHADOWS COME INTO VIEW

"There comes a stage when you stop asking if something is wrong and begin quietly asking how long it has been happening — and that realization changes everything."

Stage Three is the point on the dementia journey where something begins to feel different. Not dramatically different. Not frighteningly different. But noticeably different, different enough that people start to tilt their heads and wonder if everything is okay.

If Stage Two was a whisper, Stage Three is a low hum... persistent, noticeable, impossible to completely ignore.

Most caregivers look back and say, "This is when I knew something was happening. I didn't know what yet, but I knew something."

This is the stage where dementia starts to reveal itself, not fully, not loudly, but enough to nudge a family into awareness. Enough to begin a shift in the relationship between the person and their memory. Enough to awaken concern, confusion, and emotional complexity.

Let's walk slowly and tenderly into Stage Three, the stage where the story shifts from invisible to visible.

The First True Signs
Stage Three is known clinically as **Mild Cognitive Decline**, but don't let the word "mild" fool you. This is the stage where dementia begins to show itself in small but meaningful ways.

Symptoms often include:
- Repeating questions or stories more frequently
- Forgetting appointments or commitments
- Losing track of time or dates
- Trouble following conversations
- Difficulty with organization or planning
- Misplacing items more frequently
- Struggling to recall recent events
- Hesitating more often when searching for words

These changes still fall into a gray area, some are normal aging, some are not. **But what makes Stage Three different is the pattern**. Forgetfulness is no longer random or occasional; it becomes more consistent, more noticeable, and more disruptive.

People in this stage are usually still fully aware that something is off, and that awareness can lead to anxiety, embarrassment, or frustration.

What's Happening In The Brain
By Stage Three, the brain is no longer able to compensate fully for the damage caused by plaques, tangles, inflammation, and shrinking neural pathways.

Let's break this down in plain language.

1. The Hippocampus Begins to Struggle More Clearly
The hippocampus is responsible for new memories and short-term storage.

In Stage Three:
- It takes longer to create new memories
- It becomes easier to lose recent ones
- Retrieval becomes hit-or-miss

Imagine trying to file papers in a cabinet with drawers that sometimes jam. Sometimes the drawer opens smoothly; other times you tug and tug before it slides out.

2. Communication Between Neurons Weakens

The connections between brain cells become less efficient.

Less efficient = slower recall, slower processing, slower thinking.

3. Multitasking and Executive Function Decline

The frontal lobe, which helps with planning, logic, order, and decision-making, begins to falter.

Tasks that require:
- Sequencing
- Remembering multiple steps
- Following complex instructions
- Problem-solving

...begin to feel overwhelming.

4. The Brain's "Compensation System" Hits Its Limit

Remember in the earlier chapters how the brain rerouted signals around damaged areas?

By Stage Three, the detours are getting crowded.

The brain is working harder to stay functional.

Stage Three is when the strain begins to show.

What The Person Experiences
Most people in Stage Three are keenly aware that they are slipping.

This is often the stage where the person feels:
- Confused
- Frustrated
- Embarrassed
- Defensive
- Fearful
- Ashamed

They may start laughing off mistakes or changing the subject to hide forgetfulness. Some people become quieter, not because they don't understand, but because they don't want to reveal their struggle.

A common experience in this stage is the sudden panic of realizing you have forgotten something that shouldn't be forgettable:
- A lunch you planned
- A medical appointment
- A birthday
- A new acquaintance's name
- Directions to a familiar place

In Stage Three, these lapses feel jarring and unsettling, not just to the person, but to their loved ones.

The Emotional Complexity Of This Stage
No two people respond to Stage Three the same way.

Some become overly apologetic: "I'm so sorry, I don't know what's wrong with me."

Some become defensive: "Everyone forgets things! Stop acting like I'm losing it."

Some become avoidant: "I don't want to go. There's too much going on. I'll stay home."

Some become humorous: "You know me, always scatterbrained!" (Even if they weren't.)

Some become anxious: "What if something is wrong with me?"

This stage is emotionally charged, because it is the first time the person confronts the possibility that something serious could be happening.

Families also feel this shift:

- A daughter notices her mother repeating a conversation three times.
- A husband watches his wife forget her hair appointment, something she never did.
- A son hears his father struggle to find simple words.
- A friend notices more confusion during group gatherings.

Stage Three is not dramatic, but it is unmistakable.

Daily Life In Stage Three

People in Stage Three can still:

- Live independently
- Drive safely (most of the time)
- Work
- Participate socially
- Handle day-to-day tasks

But they often begin to:

- Create More Compensations, more notes, more lists, more reminders, more alarms
- Avoid Overwhelming Situations, "No, I don't want to go," becomes more common
- Struggle in Crowded or Noisy Environments
- Conversations overlap, sensory input overwhelms, the brain tires faster

- Take Longer to Make Decisions
- Accidentally Make Mistakes
- Paying a bill twice
- Forgetting to pay a bill
- Mixing up dates
- Leaving food out
- Misplacing keys repeatedly

The mistakes are small, but they begin to pile up.

When Families Begin to Notice
Stage Three is often the first time that loved ones say a silent version of the same sentence:

"Something isn't right."

They may not say it aloud, but they feel it.

Families start to experience:
- More worry
- More tension
- More questions
- More frustration
- More protectiveness

It's common for family members to disagree during this stage.

The overly concerned one: "We need to get her checked!"

The dismissive one: "She's just getting older. You're overreacting."

The hopeful one: "It's probably stress. She'll be fine."

The scared one: "I don't want to talk about it."

Every family has these dynamics.

Stage Three exposes them.

A Story From This Stage

My mother, Betty, had always been sharp as a tack. She was quick-witted, organized, and the kind of woman who could manage a household, stretch a dollar, and keep a calendar tighter than any smartphone app. Her mind had always been her strength, steady, reliable, and strong.

But around this stage, we began noticing little things. Small ripples on the surface.

A repeated story here.

A repeated question there.

Nothing dramatic. Nothing alarming. Just... echoes. Moments where her words circled back as if the first version had drifted away before she even realized it.

At the time, we brushed it off.

Everyone repeats stories as they get older, right?

Everyone forgets a detail or gets mixed up now and then.

Mom and Dad were living in a retirement community in Florida during these years. They kept active physically, and were socially involved, especially through the weekly bingo nights. It was their routine. Their social hour. Their contribution to the community.

Dad was the caller, the booming voice with the jokes and the charm. Mom sold the bingo cards with her warm smile and friendly chatter. It was simple work, the kind of task she could do in her sleep. For decades, she had managed all their finances: bills, budgets, checkbooks. Money was never something she struggled with.

But one evening, Dad noticed something.

As she made change for the one-dollar bingo boards, she hesitated.

Or she'd hand him the money and say softly, "Check me."

These weren't large sums.

These weren't complex calculations.

This was the kind of simple arithmetic she had done effortlessly her entire life.

And yet, she doubted herself.

It wasn't the mistake itself that worried Dad. It was the uncertainty. The second-guessing. The fact that she needed reassurance for something she had mastered fifty years earlier.

Around that same time, Dad began noticing subtle changes in her social interactions. Mom, who had always looked people in the eye when she spoke, now seemed to look away, almost past them, or through them. Her attention wasn't focused. Her gaze drifted. And during conversations, she would frequently glance toward Dad, as if searching his face for confirmation: Am I telling this right? Is this the correct detail? Am I remembering this correctly?

It was small. Gentle. Easy to overlook.

Dad thought it was odd, yes, but Stage Three is designed to look harmless. It's built on ambiguity. A moment of confusion here, a lapse in detail there. At this point, it is very easy, almost natural, to chalk everything up to normal aging.

And that's exactly what we did.

Because in Stage Three, the signs are soft.

And denial is softer still.

Looking back now, those tiny changes were the early footsteps of dementia quietly entering my mother's life. But at the time, they felt like nothing more than aging, little quirks that anyone might develop late in life.

That is the heartbreak of Stage Three:

The signs are real, but they disguise themselves as ordinary.

No one wants to imagine their loved one is losing pieces of themselves, so we explain it away. We normalize it. We reassure ourselves that everyone forgets things. Everyone gets distracted. Everyone hesitates sometimes.

We miss the early signs not because we're careless, but because we're human.

In Stage Three, dementia doesn't take away big things, it shifts small things. Eye contact. Confidence. Fluency in daily routines. The certainty they once carried so naturally. What we witnessed at bingo and in casual conversations were not failures, they were flickers, tiny signals that the brain was beginning to struggle.

Mom's hesitations with money weren't about math.

They were about processing.

They were about losing trust in her own thoughts.

They were about glimpses of confusion she couldn't yet name.

And her glances toward Dad weren't requests for approval, they were pleas for grounding. Quiet, instinctive nudges from a mind beginning to feel unsteady.

Stage Three is where families often begin to sense that something is changing, even if they don't understand what. It's the stage where caregivers start to lean in a little closer without knowing why. The stage where a loved one begins to rely on subtle cues, reassurance, and familiar faces in ways they hadn't before.

These early signs are easy to miss. Easy to excuse. Easy to forgive.

But later, when you look back, you realize these were the first gentle whispers of a journey you didn't yet recognize you were on.

And the truth is, no one ever recognizes Stage Three while they're living it.

You only understand its meaning in hindsight, when the signs make sense, when the pieces fall together, and when love helps you see what was always there, quietly unfolding.

When Medial Evaluation Becomes Possible
Stage Three is typically the earliest point when cognitive testing can reveal:

- Reduced short-term memory
- Mild decline in executive function
- Slower processing
- Word-finding difficulty
- Lower-than-expected recall

Doctors may use:

- The MoCA (Montreal Cognitive Assessment)
- The MMSE (Mini-Mental State Examination)
- Neuropsychological testing
- MRI or CT imaging

These may not confirm dementia yet, but they can show measurable decline.

The person may be diagnosed with:

- MCI (Mild Cognitive Impairment), or "Possible early dementia".

This diagnosis is frightening, but it is also a doorway to support, education, and planning.

The Caregiver's Role Begins

This is usually the stage where caregiving begins, not in a big, dramatic way, but in small supportive steps.

Caregiving at Stage Three includes:
- Gently reminding without criticizing
- Helping organize appointments
- Encouraging routines
- Simplifying tasks
- Offering support during stressful events
- Observing patterns for changes
- Encouraging evaluation (without force)

But the most important part?

Preserving the person's dignity.

They are not "losing themselves" yet.

They are aware.

They are still fully capable of love, learning, humor, creativity, and independence.

They just need more grace than they used to.

The Emotional Heart of Stage Three

This stage is emotionally charged because:

The person knows something is wrong, the family knows something is wrong, but no one wants to admit it.

It's the doorway between denial and acceptance.

It's where you begin to understand that the journey has begun, even if you're not ready to name it.

It is one of the hardest stages emotionally, because you can still see the person clearly.

They are still mostly themselves.

They are still living independently.

They are still "there."

And yet...

You begin to sense that something precious is slipping, one thread at a time.

The Transition Into Stage Four

Stage Three ends when:

- Forgetfulness becomes consistent
- Functionality becomes affected
- Tasks become overwhelming
- The person begins relying on others
- Symptoms begin interfering with daily life

Stage Four is the stage where dementia steps fully into the light, where diagnosis becomes clear, and help becomes necessary.

The shadow becomes substance.

The whisper becomes a voice.

And the journey becomes undeniable.

STAGE 4:
WHEN THE TRUTH STEPS INTO THE LIGHT

*"A diagnosis does not create the loss;
it simply confirms what your
heart has already begun to fear."*

Stage Four is where dementia finally steps out from the shadows and into clear view. It is often called **Moderate Cognitive Decline**, but to families, it becomes the moment when suspicion turns into understanding, and uncertainty turns into reality.

If Stage Three was the quiet knocking on the door, Stage Four is when the door creaks open, and dementia introduces itself.

This stage is not the most severe, not the most dramatic, not the most heartbreaking.

But it is the stage where life changes in a way that is undeniable.

It is the stage of diagnosis.

The stage of acceptance.

The stage of planning.

The stage where independence begins to wobble.

It is also the stage where the person living with dementia becomes painfully aware that something is wrong.

Let's walk carefully into this chapter, the one where understanding becomes essential and compassion becomes a daily practice.

Symptoms Become Unmistakable
In Stage Four, the symptoms increase in frequency and intensity. They are no longer random lapses, but patterns that interfere with daily life. Symptoms include:

- Forgetting important recent events
- Difficulty managing finances or paying bills
- Confusion about dates, schedules, and time
- Trouble completing familiar tasks
- Word-finding problems that disrupt conversation
- Increased forgetfulness of new information
- Becoming overwhelmed by planning or organizing
- Withdrawing from social activities
- Making more noticeable mistakes
- Signs of anxiety or depression

The person may repeat themselves more often. They may lose things daily: phones, keys, wallets, glasses, because the memory of where they placed them fades quickly.

They may struggle with multi-step tasks like:
- Cooking a meal with several steps
- Planning a route for errands
- Following instructions
- Managing medication schedules
- Balancing a checkbook

They may start asking loved ones for help more frequently, even if reluctantly. They may also begin to avoid tasks they once handled easily because dealing with them now causes frustration or embarrassment.

This is the stage where friends, extended family, neighbors, or coworkers begin noticing something's wrong. The changes are no longer subtle. They affect conversations, routines, responsibilities, and relationships.

What's Happening In the Brain
The brain changes of Stage Four are significant, and they affect several key regions. Let's break this down in simple terms.

1. The Hippocampus Is Further Damaged

This structure helps form and store new memories. By Stage Four:

- New memories fade quickly
- Recent events cannot be held long enough to transfer into long-term storage
- Conversations may be forgotten moments after they happen

This leads to repeated questions or repeated stories.

2. The Frontal Lobe Struggles

This part of the brain manages "executive function," which includes:

- Planning
- Organization
- Judgment
- Decision-making
- Multitasking

When the frontal lobe struggles, daily tasks become overwhelming. Choosing an outfit may require help. Planning a meal may feel impossible. Making decisions may cause anxiety.

3. The Brain's Processing Speed Slows Down

People in Stage Four may take longer to respond during conversations. They may pause as they search for words or struggle to follow details.

This is not stubbornness.

Not confusion.

Not disinterest.

It is the brain working harder to do what once came effortlessly.

4. Amyloid Plaques and Tau Tangles Spread

More areas of the brain are affected by:

- Plaque buildup between neurons
- Tangles interfering inside neurons

These changes disrupt communication throughout the brain, causing more noticeable cognitive decline.

The Person's Inner Experience

Stage Four can be emotionally devastating for the person living with dementia because it is often the first stage where they know something is wrong and cannot hide it anymore.

They may feel:

- Fear
- Shame
- Embarrassment
- Anxiety
- Deep sadness
- Anger
- Helplessness
- Isolation

They may say:

- "Why am I forgetting so much?"
- "I don't understand what's happening."
- "I feel confused."
- "I can't remember things anymore."
- "This isn't like me."

Many people in Stage Four try to cover up their symptoms, leading to moments of exhaustion or frustration. Others begin to withdraw socially because they don't want others to see their struggle.

The Silent Grief of Stage Four
People grieve privately:

- The loss of confidence
- The loss of control
- The loss of independence

The beginning of acknowledging the diagnosis
This is one of the most emotionally complex stages, because the person still has enough awareness to feel the weight of what is happening.

Family Members Begin to Shift Roles
Stage Four is often when families begin stepping into more active support roles, not full caregiving yet, but helpful involvement.

Common signs the family starts to notice:
- Missed appointments
- Unpaid bills
- Confusion with medications
- Difficulty managing phone calls or messages
- Getting lost on familiar routes
- Asking for help more frequently
- A sudden drop in confidence

Loved ones may begin stepping in to:
- Sort mail
- Organize calendars
- Help with finances
- Assist with errands
- Manage medications
- Supervise more
- Attend appointments together

These acts may seem small, but they mark the beginning of the caregiving journey.

The Diagnosis Often Happens In Stage Four

Most dementia diagnoses occur between Stage Three and Stage Four, but it is in Stage Four that the symptoms become clear enough to meet diagnostic criteria.

Doctors may use:
- Cognitive testing (MoCA, MMSE)
- Brain imaging (MRI, CT)
- Neuropsychological assessments
- Bloodwork to rule out other causes
- Detailed interviews with family

A diagnosis can be:
- Alzheimer's disease
- Lewy body dementia
- Vascular dementia
- Frontotemporal dementia
- Mixed dementia
- Mild Cognitive Impairment progressing to dementia

The Impact of Diagnosis

The diagnosis, though painful, often brings:

- Relief ("At least we know what's happening.")
- Clarity ("We have a direction now.")
- Guidance ("What do we do next?")
- A plan ("We can prepare for what's coming.")

Family members often begin researching, reading, asking questions, and building a support system.

For the person with dementia, the diagnosis is a moment of reality that may trigger:

- Depression
- Anxiety
- Acceptance
- Avoidance
- Denial

Everyone responds differently.

Daily Life In Stage Four

In Stage Four, independence still exists but begins to require maintenance and supervision.

Tasks People Still Handle Independently:

- Basic self-care
- Simple meals
- Simple household tasks
- Familiar routines
- Light social interaction

Tasks That Become Challenging

- Managing bills
- Understanding complex instructions
- Learning new technologies
- Planning trips or events
- Managing medications
- Cooking multi-step meals
- Shopping alone
- Driving safely

Mistakes become more noticeable.

Social Situations Become More Difficult

Crowds, noise, or rapid conversations may overwhelm them. They may smile and pretend to follow along, but their mind may be struggling to keep up.

Emotional Responses Increase

People may cry more easily.

Become frustrated quickly.

Lose patience with themselves.

Experience feelings of failure or embarrassment.

A Story From This Stage

In my parents' retirement years, they lived a rhythm that suited them perfectly: six months of warm Florida sunshine in their RV, and six months with me in North Carolina. It was a simple pattern, predictable and comforting. Their doctors, their prescriptions, their routines, those were all anchored in Florida. When they stayed with me, it was never for medical reasons. It was just part of the life they enjoyed.

But in the summer of 2014, everything shifted.

Mom came down with what seemed like a stubborn cold, nothing more than a nuisance at first. When it worsened and settled into her lungs, turning into pneumonia, she had no choice but to see my doctor in North Carolina. It felt strange, taking her outside of her usual medical world, but necessary. None of us had any reason to think this visit would become a turning point in our lives.

During her treatment and follow-up scans, the doctor found a spot on her lung.

A small shadow.

A maybe.

A question no one wants to ask.

Further testing confirmed it: lung cancer.

Suddenly, the life they had built, the RV winters, the road trips, the freedom, became uncertain. Treatment would require consistency. Doctors. Specialists. Regular appointments. So, my parents made the difficult decision to give up their RV in Florida and move in with me full-time, choosing stability and family support over the independence they had always treasured.

Shortly after the diagnosis, Dad and I planned a long weekend trip back to Florida to clean out the RV, sell it, and bring home their belongings. It seemed simple, logistical. Mom would stay behind, it made practical sense. If she stayed home, we had more room in the car to haul items. Leaving her alone for a few days wasn't even a concern. She had lived independently her whole life. At that point, we weren't even whispering the word Alzheimer's. We didn't know to look for signs. We didn't know a storm was slowly forming.

Just to give her a little company in the evenings, we asked my nephew, Matthew, to stay overnight with her. Not to supervise. Not to oversee anything. Just to be a warm body in the house, someone she could chat with before bed. We didn't place responsibility on him because we truly believed she didn't require any.

Dad handled the medications in their daily life, not out of necessity, but habit. He liked the routine. He filled the weekly pill organizer and handed the pills out each day. So, before we left, he placed her weekly pill dispenser on the kitchen counter. Monday through Sunday, neatly labeled.

We assumed she would take Friday's pills on Friday, Saturday's pills on Saturday.

It was a perfectly reasonable assumption, until it wasn't.

When we returned four days later, something felt off. The pill organizer was empty. Completely empty.

Seven days of medications consumed in four days.

Mom had no explanation. She didn't argue, didn't deny, didn't apologize. She simply... moved on, as if nothing unusual had happened. But to us, something inside the room shifted. Suddenly, the air felt heavier. The pieces that didn't previously make sense now quietly rearranged themselves.

Looking back, the signs were there.

She couldn't remember whether she'd taken her pills.

She couldn't connect the day of the week to the correct compartment in the organizer.

And when in doubt... she took more.

It was luck, pure grace, that none of her medications were dangerous in excess. But it could have ended very differently.

The realization hit us with quiet force: she needed oversight.

This wasn't stubbornness.

This wasn't forgetfulness in the harmless sense.

This was something deeper. Something cognitive. Something we didn't yet understand.

But at the time, our entire focus was on lung cancer: appointments, treatment plans, fear of the unknown. We hadn't even begun to grasp that another, more invisible disease was unfolding beneath the surface.

That weekend was the first time we were confronted with the truth: Mom's mind was slipping in ways we hadn't recognized. And for the first time, the question we hadn't dared to ask began whispering its way into our thoughts.

That moment with the pill organizer was more than a mishap, it was the quiet doorway into Stage Four. It was the stage of almost: almost independent, almost aware, almost the same as before... until she wasn't.

Stage Four is subtle.

It doesn't shout.

It doesn't announce itself.

It shows up in the small cracks of everyday life, the questions repeated, the items misplaced, the routines forgotten, the mistakes rationalized away.

And because the changes are gradual, families often miss them. We did.

We told ourselves she was tired. Distracted. Under stress from her cancer diagnosis. But Stage Four had already begun rewriting the rules, and we just hadn't learned to read the signs yet.

It is the stage where loved ones still appear capable... right up until they aren't.

The stage where independence flickers, not gone, but unreliable.

The stage where caregivers begin to realize that something is wrong, even if they can't name it yet.

Looking back, the empty pill organizer wasn't a crisis, it was a message.

A gentle warning.

A moment of truth delivered through something so ordinary it could easily have been ignored.

It was the day we unknowingly crossed into unfamiliar territory.

The day we realized she needed us in ways we hadn't anticipated.

The day we began paying closer attention.

The day Alzheimer's whispered its first unmistakable clue.

Stage Four is the beginning of awareness.

Not full recognition, not diagnosis, but awareness.

And for our family, that awareness began with seven empty compartments and a truth we weren't yet ready to understand.

The Caregiver's New Role
In Stage Four, caregivers begin transitioning from "family" to "support system."

Not fully, not overwhelmingly, but gently.

Caregiving responsibilities might include:
- Simplifying tasks
- Offering supportive reminders
- Attending appointments together
- Organizing paperwork
- Assisting with transportation
- Helping manage medications
- Providing emotional reassurance
- Caregivers also begin to grieve

They grieve:
- The first visible losses
- The shift in roles
- The fear of what's coming
- The pain of watching someone struggle

But they also learn new strengths:
- Patience
- Compassion
- Flexibility
- Advocacy
- Presence

Stage Four is where caregivers start to grow in ways they never asked to, but rise to, out of love.

The Importance of Routine and Support

Routine becomes comforting in Stage Four.

Predictability helps reduce anxiety.

Helpful strategies include:
- Keeping a consistent daily schedule
- Simplifying the home environment
- Reducing clutter
- Keeping important items in the same place
- Using calendars, whiteboards, or reminders
- Encouraging safe independence
- Limiting overwhelming situations
- Support Begins to Matter

Stage Four is an important time to build a support system:
- Support groups
- Memory clinics
- Caregiver education
- Community programs
- Legal planning
- Financial planning
- Counseling

These tools help pave the road for the stages ahead.

The Transition Into Stage Five

Stage Four transitions into Stage Five when:

- The person begins needing help with daily living
- Confusion increases
- Independence declines more noticeably
- New memories fade quickly
- Orientation to time and place becomes inconsistent
- The ability to choose appropriate clothing declines
- Daily tasks become overwhelming

Stage Five is the beginning of moderately severe cognitive decline, a stage where caregiving becomes a daily responsibility, not just an occasional support.

But Stage Four?

This is the stage of **realization**.

The stage of **diagnosis**.

The stage of **preparation**.

The stage where love deepens in new, painful, beautiful ways.

It is the stage where dementia stops being a possibility and becomes a reality, but a reality surrounded by compassion, support, and dignity.

STAGE 5:
WHEN HELP BECOMES NECESSARY

"The first time you must step in and do what they once did with ease, you feel the shift — not just in responsibility, but in the shape of your relationship."

Stage Five is the turning point of dementia.

Not the beginning, and certainly not the end, but the moment when the disease becomes impossible to ignore. This is the stage where independence begins to slip through a person's hands, not all at once, but piece by piece, task by task, day by day.

If Stage Four was recognition, Stage Five is acceptance.

If Stage Four was the diagnosis, Stage Five is the adjustment.

If Stage Four was noticing changes, Stage Five is responding to them.

The person you love is still very much here, still present, still aware, still capable of joy and humor and connection, but they need help now. Not suggestions. Not reminders. Not occasional support.

Actual, daily assistance.

This is the stage where caregivers become essential.

Let's gently step into Stage Five together, with tenderness for the person living through it and compassion for the caregiver learning how to navigate an ever-changing world.

The Defining Characteristic of Stage Five: Loss of Independence

Stage Five: **Moderately Severe Cognitive Decline**, is the stage where dementia meaningfully interferes with daily living.

This is not just forgetting appointments or repeating questions.

This is needing help to function.

Stage Five is diagnosed when a person can no longer manage one or more Activities of Daily Living (ADLs) without assistance:
- Dressing
- Bathing
- Choosing appropriate clothing
- Grooming
- Managing hygiene
- Preparing meals

- Managing medication
- Navigating safely
- Handling basic household responsibilities

The person can still feed themselves, use the bathroom with minimal assistance, and participate in many routines, but the loss of independence becomes clear.

Symptoms of Stage Five

Common cognitive and functional symptoms include:

- Forgetting their address
- Forgetting where they live (but not the city)
- Forgetting important personal details
- Needing help choosing clothing
- Putting clothes on in the wrong order
- Wearing inappropriate clothing for the weather
- Forgetting to bathe unless prompted
- Forgetting to eat regularly
- Difficulty preparing food
- Trouble using appliances safely
- Inability to manage medications
- Forgetting names of grandchildren or extended family
- Confusion about the date, time, or season
- Becoming overwhelmed by simple tasks
- Significant short-term memory loss

- Difficulty learning new information
- Loss of financial judgment

Despite these losses, the person usually:
- Knows their own name
- Knows the names of close family
- Remembers childhood memories vividly
- Recognizes familiar faces
- Enjoys music, conversations, and routines
- Participates in social interactions

This is the stage where long-term memories strengthen emotionally, even as short-term memories fade almost instantly.

What's Happening In The Brain

By Stage Five, the brain has sustained substantial damage. Here's what's happening, explained simply.

1. The Hippocampus Is Severely Compromised

This region, responsible for forming new memories, is one of the first to deteriorate in dementia. By Stage Five:
- New memories last minutes or seconds
- Recent conversations vanish quickly
- Learning new skills becomes nearly impossible

2. The Parietal Lobe Is Affected

This part of the brain helps with:

- Dressing
- Spatial awareness
- Understanding directions
- Following sequences

Damage here explains why a person may put a shirt on backward or struggle with simple, step-by-step tasks.

3. The Temporal Lobe Declines

This region manages:

- Language
- Understanding speech
- Recognizing faces
- Storing memories

As it deteriorates, word-finding issues increase and misunderstandings become more frequent.

4. The Frontal Lobe Loses More Function

This region controls:

- Judgment
- Problem-solving
- Planning
- Impulse control

This is why a person might:
- Give away money
- Leave the stove on
- Wander outside
- Argue more than usual

5. Emotional Memory Remains Strong
Even as cognitive function declines, the amygdala
(the brain's emotional center) remains active. The
person may not remember your name, but they will
remember:
- Your voice
- Your tone
- Your kindness
- Your touch

They remember how you make them feel, even when
they cannot recall other details.

The Person's Inner Experience
This is one of the most emotionally challenging
stages for the person living with dementia. Why?

Because they still understand enough to know
they're losing parts of themselves.

They may say things like:
- "I can't remember anything anymore."
- "I feel stupid."
- "Why is this happening to me?"

- "I hate this."
- "What's wrong with me?"

Shame is common.

Fear is common.

Anger is common.

Sadness is common.

In Stage Five, the person often becomes painfully aware of their limitations, yet unable to overcome them alone.

Imagine forgetting how to put on your clothes.

Imagine forgetting how to start the shower.

Imagine forgetting what month it is.

Imagine forgetting which side of the house your bedroom is on.

This creates an emotional landscape filled with:
- Frustration
- Anxiety
- Panic
- Tears
- Withdrawal
- Depression

And yet... there is also beauty.

People in Stage Five still love deeply.

They still laugh.

They still enjoy music, affection, stories, prayer, and familiar routines.

They still express gratitude, tenderness, humor, and childlike joy.

They are losing abilities, not their humanity.

What Daily Life Looks Like In Stage Five
Life in this stage shifts dramatically. Let's explore.

1. Dressing Challenges
A common sign of Stage Five is difficulty choosing appropriate clothing.

Examples:
- Wearing pajamas to the store
- Wearing winter clothing on a hot day
- Wearing three layers of shirts but no pants
- Trying to put both legs in one pant hole
- Forgetting how to button or zip

They need guidance, not criticism.

2. Hygiene Requires Assistance

Not because they don't want to be clean, but because:

- They forget the steps
- They forget when they last bathed
- They feel overwhelmed
- They fear slipping
- They lose track of time

Gentle prompting becomes necessary.

3. Eating Becomes Disorganized

People may:

- Forget to eat
- Forget they ate
- Leave food out
- Eat only snacks because cooking feels too complex
- Struggle to follow multi-step cooking tasks

Providing simple meals and steady routines helps.

4. Finances Are No Longer Safe

By Stage Five, the person:

- Cannot manage money safely
- Forgets to pay bills
- Falls for scams
- Loses track of spending
- Gives away money impulsively

Caregivers MUST take over financial management.

5. Social Withdrawal Begins

People may avoid gatherings because:

- They can't follow fast conversations
- Noise overwhelms them
- They feel embarrassed
- They fear making mistakes

But gentle, simple social interaction is still beneficial.

6. Wandering May Begin

Confusion increases. They may:

- Walk out the door
- Forget where they were going
- Get lost in familiar places

Safety becomes a critical concern.

A Story From This Stage

In December of 2014, I planned a cruise for Mom, Dad, my brother Dave, and my sister-in-law, Marie. It felt like the perfect family adventure, a chance to make happy memories while Mom was still functioning well enough to enjoy them. She was forgetful, yes, but still largely herself. Still able to travel. Still able to laugh. Still able to be part of the fun.

We packed days in advance. Mom and Dad's suitcase sat in the loft outside their bedroom, my home office turned staging area for every family trip we ever took. I could hear Mom in the evenings calling up the stairs:

"Did I pack a nightgown?"

And Dad, patient as always, would reassure her:

"Yes, Betty. You have everything you need."

Five minutes later, she'd quietly slip upstairs, retrieve another nightgown, and tuck it into the suitcase. At first it was endearing. Cute, even. But as the night went on, we realized the suitcase was getting fuller… and fuller… and fuller. Not with essentials, but with whatever items temporarily soothed her anxiety.

Dad's solution was simple but effective: he locked the suitcase.

That lock wasn't about control; it was about calm. When Mom felt compelled to pack yet another item, Dad could gently remind her:

"It's already in there. You're all set."

It became our first real glimpse of obsessional behavior, the looping thoughts, the need for reassurance, the comfort of repetition.

Once we were on the cruise, the next clue arrived. I hadn't noticed it at first. In fact, it took Marie quietly pulling me aside and whispering, "Josh... we need to get her to wear something else."

That's when I finally saw it.

Mom was wearing a Halloween sweater she'd picked up at Goodwill: bright orange pumpkins, sparkly stitching, and sleeves that had become thin from wear. It was December. On a cruise. Surrounded by people wearing tropical florals and sundresses. And there she was, proudly sporting Halloween in the Caribbean.

Every morning Dad and I would gently suggest something different. Another sweater. A blouse. Anything. But by midday she'd be wearing the Halloween sweater again.

Finally, we "disappeared" it.

And just like that, no fight, no confusion, her wardrobe rotated normally again. It was our first lesson that in dementia, out of sight is often out of mind.

That pattern continued at home. She'd wear the same outfit for days until we quietly removed it from her room. Then, magically, variety returned. It wasn't stubbornness. It was comfort. Familiarity. Routine.

But the cruise was only the beginning.

In February 2017, I had a conference at the Disneyland Hotel in California, and I decided to take Mom and Dad along. I had enough Southwest points to cover the flights, and the idea of giving them one last big adventure together felt right.

Mobility wasn't an issue, Mom was in a wheelchair by then, but her spirit was good, and Disneyland had always been a place of magic for our family.

We spent several days together in the park before my conference began. When the day of my sessions arrived, I stayed at the hotel while Mom and Dad headed into Disneyland on their own. Dad pushed the wheelchair; Mom hummed happily; and the two of them set off like teenagers on a date.

They stopped for lunch in Frontierland. Dad went to grab food while Mom waited in her wheelchair at the table. When he returned, she stood up and announced she needed to use the restroom. Dad pointed it out, it was about 50 yards away, she made it there and back without any trouble.

They ate their lunch. They relaxed. It felt like a normal moment, a comfortable rhythm.

Then Mom said she needed the restroom again.

Dad pointed to the same place. She nodded and walked off, mobile enough to manage it. He trusted the moment. Why wouldn't he? She had literally just done this thirty minutes earlier.

But this time… she didn't come back.

Fifteen minutes passed.

Then twenty.

Then thirty.

Dad couldn't leave the table, the wheelchair, the food, the belongings were all in his care, so he flagged down a Disney security guard.

She wasn't in the restroom.

She wasn't in Frontierland.

She was gone.

Disney immediately began a park-wide search. They notified local authorities. The Orange County Police Department issued a Silver Alert. My mother wasn't just missing; she was legally missing.

Meanwhile, I was sitting in a conference session, blissfully unaware, until I received a text from Dad that began:

"You're going to kill me, but…"

My heart dropped.

Thankfully, the Disneyland Hotel is a quick walk to the park. I ran, literally ran, to the main entrance. Police officers were already there, calm but alert, reassuring me:

"We're watching every exit. She cannot leave the park. We will find her."

Dad was taken to City Hall to wait. The security guard and I continued searching. I remember scanning every face, every bench, every line, praying for one familiar silhouette.

And then, I turned a corner onto Main Street and saw the security guard again. He was walking toward me… smiling.

He'd found her.

Mom was standing in the bakery on Main Street, content, unbothered, and absolutely thrilled to have found her way to the sweets. She had walked out of the restroom, turned the opposite direction, wandered into Fantasyland, and then simply followed whichever whim pulled her next.

Hours passed. She never looked distressed. Never looked lost. Never asked for help. To Disney Cast Members, she was just another happy older woman enjoying the park.

What saved her that day wasn't awareness.

It was joy.

She was too blissful to seem out of place.

Her lanyard, listing her name, memory condition, and our phone numbers, hung around her neck. It was meant for emergencies, for moments when she looked scared or confused. But she never triggered concern, because she never felt concerned.

After that, everything changed.

We understood, deeply, painfully, how quickly short-term memory could disappear. She had used that restroom successfully minutes earlier. Yet on her second visit, she walked out, turned left instead of right, and her world instantly became unanchored.

She didn't forget the restroom.

She forgot the moment.

She forgot the sequence.

She forgot the responsibility to return.

And she wandered into a world that no longer held a map for her.

That day at Disneyland became one of the defining moments of Stage Five for us. It was the day we truly understood the fragile balance dementia creates, where a person can appear capable one moment and become profoundly lost the next. Stage Five is unpredictable like that. It's the stage where independence flickers: sometimes bright, sometimes dim, never reliable.

In the earlier stages, misplacing a sweater or packing too many nightgowns is frustrating, but manageable. But getting lost in a theme park, the same restroom she had just navigated successfully? That is when the stakes change. When you realize dementia is not just forgetfulness, it is disorientation wrapped in innocence.

It's the stage where caregivers begin to fear the moments they cannot control.

The moments when a wrong turn becomes a crisis.

The moments when something familiar suddenly becomes foreign.

The moments when a simple bathroom break becomes a Silver Alert.

But Stage Five also teaches something beautifully heartbreaking:

They aren't wandering away from you.

They are wandering into the world as they now see it, without maps, without anchors, without time.

Mom didn't disappear that day because she was careless.

She disappeared because dementia had already begun to erase the pathways that lead a person back.

And yet… she was happy.

She was safe.

She was found.

That twisting emotional cocktail, fear and relief, grief and gratitude, is what defines Stage Five. It's the stage where you begin to realize your role is shifting from helper to guardian. From companion to protector. From someone who walks beside your loved one… to someone who must sometimes walk ahead and clear the path for them.

Stage Five is the beginning of letting go of the illusion of control.

It's the beginning of loving someone enough to change the rules, the routines, the expectations.

It's the beginning of learning that independence can disappear in an instant and reappear just as fast.

It's the stage where love becomes vigilant and caregiving becomes instinct and every moment becomes both a gift and a warning.

And it's the stage that prepares your heart, slowly and painfully, for the journey still ahead.

The Caregiver's Role In Stage Five
Caregiving becomes a daily responsibility now.

Not heavy, not overwhelming yet, but essential.

Needs caregivers should begin providing:

1. Help with Dressing
- Offer choices
- Keep clothing simple
- Lay outfits out in order
- Avoid complicated fasteners

2. Help with Hygiene
- Establish routines like "Shower every morning before breakfast."
- Keep supplies where they are easy to see.
- Assist without rushing or judging.

3. Safety Supervision
The house may need:
- Door alarms
- Stove safety devices
- Clear walkways
- Labels on rooms
- Nightlights
- Hidden car keys

4. Emotional Support

- Be patient.
- Use a gentle tone.
- Validate their feelings.

5. Medication Management

The person can no longer handle this independently.

6. Financial Management

Bills, accounts, credit cards, insurance, all need to be the caregiver responsibility now.

7. Consistent Routines

Routines reduce:

- Anxiety
- Confusion
- Outbursts
- Wandering

Behavioral Changes In Stage Five

As cognitive function declines, the person may experience:

- Irritability
- Mood swings
- Anxiety
- Accusations ("Someone stole my keys!")
- Frustration
- Resistance to help
- Emotional outbursts
- Clinging or dependence

These behaviors are symptoms, not personality flaws.

Not stubbornness.

Not intentional.

They are signals of fear, confusion, and frustration.

The Beauty That Remains

Even with these losses, Stage Five is filled with meaningful moments:

- The person still recognizes loved ones
- They can express love and gratitude
- They can enjoy activities
- They can laugh, sing, dance
- They can reminisce
- They can cherish simple joys

In many ways, Stage Five becomes a stage of emotional intimacy, a time when relationships deepen through vulnerability, tenderness, and presence.

The Transition Into Stage Six

Stage Five ends when the person:

- Can no longer bathe or dress independently
- Cannot manage toileting needs without help
- Loses track of close family members
- Struggles with nighttime confusion
- Shows significant behavioral changes
- Becomes unable to control impulses
- Needs full assistance with daily life

Stage Six is the stage of severe cognitive decline, where caregiving becomes full-time and profound.

But Stage Five?

This is the stage of caregiving foundations.

This is the stage where compassion expands.

This is the stage where love becomes an action, daily, patient, deliberate.

STAGE 6:
WHEN THE WORLD BECOMES UNCERTAIN

"When memory fades and independence disappears, love is asked to carry more than it ever imagined, and somehow, it does."

Stage Six is one of the most difficult chapters on the dementia journey. Not because love disappears, or connection disappears, or the person disappears, but because the disease begins to affect nearly every part of life. Memory becomes fragile. Identity becomes inconsistent. Familiar routines become confusing, and daily care becomes essential.

This is the stage of **Severe Cognitive Decline**.

The stage where caregivers become lifelines.

The stage where the person living with dementia enters a world that feels unpredictable, shifting, and often frightening.

Yet even in this stage, there is beauty, quiet beauty, subtle beauty, the kind that hides in small moments: the squeeze of a hand, a sudden smile, the comfort of music, the recognition in their eyes when you enter the room.

Stage Six is heartbreaking, yes. But it is also sacred.

Let's walk into it gently.

What Defines Stage Six?
Stage Six is marked by major memory loss, increasing confusion, and significant decline in the ability to perform daily activities.

Key characteristics include:

- Forgetting the names of close family members
- Forgetting major parts of their personal history
- Needing help with bathing, dressing, toileting, and grooming
- Difficulty communicating
- Increased anxiety and agitation
- Sleep disturbances and "sundowning"
- Wandering or pacing
- Hallucinations or delusions
- Emotional unpredictability
- Loss of impulse control
- Repetitive behaviors or speech
- Difficulty recognizing familiar places
- Loss of bladder or bowel control (in many cases)

At this stage, the disease is no longer subtle or intermittent.

It is constant and pervasive.

The brain is struggling to interpret the world.

But always remember:

Inside this stage, the emotional heart still beats strongly.

Their ability to feel love, comfort, pain, fear, safety, joy, and peace remains.

What's Happening In the Brain?
Stage Six involves significant damage to several key areas of the brain.

Let's break this down in simple terms:

1. The Hippocampus Is Severely Damaged
This affects:

- New memory formation
- Orientation to time and place
- The ability to remember people

This is why the person may look at their adult child and say: "Are you my sister?" or "How long have I known you?"

They may still feel love but cannot place the relationship.

2. The Parietal Lobe Weakens Further

This disrupts:

- Dressing
- Bathing
- Spatial awareness
- Recognizing objects
- Body orientation

This explains why a person may:

- Put pants on their arms
- Use toothpaste as lotion
- Fail to notice when clothing is inside-out
- Need help in the bathroom

3. The Temporal Lobe Deteriorates

This affects:

- Language comprehension
- Speech
- Recognition of familiar faces and sounds

The person may:

- Struggle to form complete sentences
- Use the wrong words
- Speak less overall
- Fail to recognize even close family members at times

4. The Frontal Lobe Declines Significantly

This impacts:

- Behavior
- Emotion regulation
- Judgment
- Social control

This can lead to:

- Impulsive behavior
- Disinhibition
- Emotional outbursts
- Increased frustration
- Accusations of theft or wrongdoing
- Paranoia

5. The Occipital Lobe May Become Involved

This affects:

- Visual processing
- Depth perception
- Interpretation of shadows

This is why hallucinations sometimes emerge, especially in Lewy body dementia.

What This Means Emotionally

The person is not "choosing" these behaviors.

They are not "being difficult."

They are losing the ability to interpret their world accurately.

Their reactions are defensive, not deliberate.

The Person's Inner World In Stage Six
This stage can feel confusing, frightening, and disorienting for the person living with dementia.

They may experience:
- Sudden fear with no clear cause
- Confusion about where they are
- Panic when left alone
- Anxiety during personal care
- Misinterpretation of normal events
- Difficulty understanding language
- Overwhelm in noisy or chaotic environments

Yet they can also experience:
- Comfort from a familiar voice
- Peace from gentle touch
- Joy from music or memories
- Laughter from simple humor
- Connection through eye contact
- Safety through routine

Recognition Becomes Emotional, Not Cognitive

Even if they can't remember your name, they remember you emotionally.

They may not know who you are, but they know who you are to them.

Your presence calms them.

Your voice reassures them.

Your routines feel safe.

Your love feels familiar.

This is one of the miracles of Stage Six:

Love remains accessible even when memory does not.

Daily Life In Stage Six

Daily life changes dramatically at this stage. Let's explore the major challenges.

1. Dressing Requires Full Assistance

The person may:

- Forget how to dress
- Put clothes on upside-down
- Layer multiple garments
- Forget to change clothes
- Resist help out of embarrassment or fear

Caregiver strategies:

- Lay clothing out in order
- Choose simple, comfortable outfits
- Use adaptive clothing (Velcro, elastic waistbands)
- Maintain gentle, calm communication
- Respect their dignity, always

2. Bathing and Hygiene Become Difficult

People may resist bathing due to:

- Fear of falling
- Discomfort with water
- Feeling cold
- Embarrassment
- Misunderstanding the process

Caregiver strategies:

- Use warm, comfortable water
- Keep the bathroom warm
- Use a handheld shower
- Provide calm explanations
- Maintain privacy as much as possible
- Celebrate small successes

3. Toileting and Incontinence

Incontinence can emerge due to:

- Confusion about bodily cues
- Slower signaling between the brain and body
- Difficulty locating the bathroom
- Trouble undressing in time

Caregiver strategies:

- Establish regular bathroom schedules
- Use clear signs or labels
- Keep the path well-lit
- Use protective garments when needed
- NEVER shame or ridicule

Loss of continence is one of the hardest emotional losses.

Compassion must be the anchor.

4. Eating and Nutrition

People in Stage Six may:

- Forget to eat
- Forget how to use utensils
- Become distracted by the environment
- Struggle to chew or swallow

Caregiver strategies:

- Offer small, frequent meals
- Use finger foods
- Limit distractions
- Provide verbal cues: "Take a bite"
- Avoid rushing
- Use smoothies or soft foods if needed

5. Nighttime Confusion (Sundowning)

This stage often includes:

- Restlessness in the late afternoon/evening
- Increased agitation
- Difficulty sleeping
- Pacing or wandering
- Heightened fear or paranoia

This is **not misbehavior**, it is neurological.

Caregiver strategies:

- Keep evenings calm and predictable
- Dim lights slowly (never suddenly)
- Avoid caffeine and sugar late in the day
- Offer soothing activities or music
- Maintain a regular sleep schedule
- Use nightlights to prevent disorientation

6. Hallucinations and Delusions

In Stage Six, misinterpretations are common:

- Shadows may look like figures
- Reflections may look like strangers
- Loud noises may trigger fear
- They may believe someone stole their belongings

Caregiver strategies:

- Do not argue
- Validate feelings ("I can see why you're upset")
- Reassure and redirect
- Reduce visual clutter
- Increase lighting to minimize shadows

A Story From Stage Six

I took Mom and Dad to Disney World in November of 2019. At that point in her dementia journey, Mom was still mostly independent in her personal care. She wore Depends, which helped with any urgency or unexpected accidents, but up until then she had always managed everything on her own. It made her feel dignified. It made us feel like we still had time before things became more complicated.

That morning, we were entering Animal Kingdom: bright sunshine, crowds spilling through the turnstiles, music playing overhead. We hadn't been inside the park more than a couple minutes when Mom said she needed to use the restroom. No problem. We walked her to the nearest women's restroom just inside the entrance.

"Go ahead, Mom. We'll be right out here," I told her.

She nodded and went inside.

And then... we waited.

And waited.

And waited.

At first, Dad and I joked about the two of us standing outside a women's restroom at Disney World like a pair of lost tourists. But after a few more minutes passed, the laughter stopped. Concern settled in. There we were, two men, completely helpless, unable to go in and see if she was okay.

We finally asked a woman walking in if she could check on her. She agreed and disappeared inside. A minute later she came back out and said, "She told me she's fine."

But something in my gut said she wasn't fine.

More minutes passed, each one heavier than the last. There's a certain feeling caregivers know all too well, that moment when you sense the line between independence and vulnerability has quietly shifted.

When Mom finally came out, everything in me twisted.

Her Depends was gone.

Her pants were inside out.

She was soiled, confused, and disoriented, embarrassed but trying to hold herself together.

My heart broke and tightened at the same time. We had an extra Depends in the backpack, but no extra clothing. This wasn't just an accident. This was a sign. A turning point. One of those moments you remember because afterward, nothing is quite the same.

It was the first time we realized that certain environments, especially busy, unfamiliar restrooms, were becoming too overwhelming for her to navigate alone. The stalls, the noise, the locks, the steps, the sequence of what to do, it was too much. Too confusing. Too easy to get lost in.

And there we were, powerless to help her in a space where only she was allowed to go.

Later that morning, a Disney Cast Member gently told us about the companion restrooms, private, single-use restrooms designed for guests who needed assistance. Places where one of us could go in with her, help her with clothing, make sure she was clean and safe, and maintain dignity instead of losing it.

From that moment on, companion restrooms became our lifeline.

It was a small shift in the grand scheme of caregiving, but emotionally, it was huge. It was the day we realized Mom could no longer manage certain bathroom situations independently. The day we accepted that her dementia had quietly moved into a new stage. The day we learned that support wasn't just helpful, it was necessary.

That moment in the Animal Kingdom restroom wasn't about embarrassment.

It was about awareness.

It was about transition.

It was about learning to protect her dignity in a world that no longer made sense to her.

And like so many moments in Stage Six, it was the place where love became a little more hands-on, a little more proactive, and a lot more tender.

Looking back, that morning at Disney World was more than just an accident in a restroom. It was a turning point in my mother's dementia journey, and in ours as her caregivers. Stage Six doesn't arrive with fanfare. There's no announcement, no clear line dividing "before" and "after." Instead, it comes to you in moments like that one: small, painful awakenings disguised as everyday mishaps.

In Stage Six, the world becomes harder for the person you love. Routines they once handled effortlessly now require step-by-step guidance. Familiar places become confusing. Private tasks become overwhelming. And as a caregiver, you begin to step deeper into their world, not because you want to, but because they need you to.

That day in Animal Kingdom forced me to see something I had been trying not to admit: Mom was losing another layer of independence. And with every layer she lost, we had to learn a new way to support her. It wasn't about taking over, it was about taking care. It was about holding onto her dignity when she no longer had the ability to protect it herself.

Stage Six teaches caregivers that love becomes more physical, more present, more intentional. It's the stage where you start assisting with things you once considered private. The stage where you realize that offering help isn't stripping someone of independence, it's giving them safety. It's giving them comfort. It's giving them grace.

That day reminded me that caregiving is not just about meeting needs. It's about seeing the person beneath the symptoms, beneath the confusion, beneath the decline. It's about staying tender even when the moments are hard. It's about accepting that the journey is changing again and choosing to meet that change with compassion rather than fear.

Stage Six asks caregivers to step deeper into love.

And that morning at Disney was the moment we took that step.

The Caregiver's Role In Stage Six
This is when caregiving becomes demanding, physically, emotionally, mentally, spiritually.

Caregivers must provide:
- Full assistance with dressing
- Full assistance with bathing
- Full assistance with toileting
- Medication management

- Meal preparation and monitoring
- Constant supervision for safety
- Emotional reassurance
- Gentle redirection
- Management of behavioral symptoms
- Stability during confusion
- Comfort during fear

Caregivers become:
- Nurses
- Counselors
- Protectors
- Advocates
- Translators of a confusing world
- Anchors in the storm

But Stage Six is also when caregivers begin to experience:
- Exhaustion
- Grief
- Guilt
- Frustration
- Isolation
- Physical strain
- Emotional heaviness
- Deep love

No one should walk Stage Six alone.

Support becomes essential.

What Helps Most In This Stage
Routine:

- Routine reduces fear.
- Repetition becomes comfort.

Visual cues:

- Labels, signs, photos and simple instructions help orient the person.

Calm tone:

- Tone matters more than words.

Gentle redirection:

- Arguing makes confusion worse.

Music:

- Music accesses memories that language cannot reach.

Touch:

- A warm hand can soothe fear more effectively than a long explanation.

Validation:

- Instead of saying "That's not real," say: "I'm here. You're safe."

Lights:

- Good lighting reduces hallucinations.

Family education:

- Understanding the disease reduces conflict.

The Beauty That Still Remains

Even in the midst of decline, beauty remains:

- A smile
- A laugh
- A gleam of recognition
- A sudden memory from childhood
- A whispered prayer
- A moment of clarity
- A peaceful afternoon nap
- A gentle dance in the kitchen
- A familiar song that brings tears
- A hand that squeezes yours

Stage Six is a different kind of love story; slower, quieter, more fragile, but also more profound.

This stage teaches caregivers something sacred:
- Presence is more powerful than perfection.
- Connection is more powerful than cognition.
- Love is more powerful than memory.

The Transition Into Stage Seven
Stage Six transitions into Stage Seven when:
- Speech becomes extremely limited
- Walking becomes difficult or impossible
- Swallowing becomes impaired
- The person becomes largely dependent
- Awareness of surroundings fades
- Physical decline accelerates

Stage Seven is the final stage, a stage of deep vulnerability, profound tenderness, and sacred care.

But Stage Six, this chapter, is where the heart learns to love without conditions, without expectations, without needing anything in return.

It is a stage where love speaks through touch, presence, tone, music, prayer, and patience.

STAGE 7: WALKING THEM HOME

"When words fall away and recognition grows thin, what remains is not knowledge, but the quiet, steady presence of love."

Stage Seven is where the dementia journey becomes both the hardest and, in many ways, the most sacred. It is the stage of **Very Severe Cognitive Decline**, and it marks the final chapter of a long and difficult path, a chapter where the body, mind, and spirit begin to slow down in preparation for life's final transition.

In this stage, the person requires total care. Speech fades, mobility fades, swallowing becomes challenging, and awareness becomes profoundly limited. But even as abilities fall away one by one, the core of the person remains; their humanity, their dignity, and their capacity to feel love and comfort.

This chapter is not about loss alone.

It is about presence.

It is about compassion.

It is about the sacred act of caring for someone in their most vulnerable state.

And it is about the extraordinary love that endures even when memory, words, and independence no longer remain.

Let's step into Stage Seven with reverence and gentleness.

What Defines Stage Seven?
Stage Seven is marked by significant physical, cognitive, and communication decline.

Key characteristics include:
- Loss of the ability to speak (or speaking only a few words)
- Loss of ability to walk or sit up without support
- Loss of ability to hold up the head
- Loss of the ability to smile or show facial expressions consistently
- Loss of bladder and bowel control
- Difficulty swallowing (dysphagia)
- High risk of aspiration (food or liquid entering the lungs)
- Vulnerability to infections, especially pneumonia
- Extended sleeping or minimal wakefulness
- Limited awareness of surroundings

- Weight loss and weakened muscles
- Total dependence for all daily living activities

Despite all of this, the person may still show:
- Recognition in their eyes
- A squeeze of the hand
- A peaceful sigh
- A moment of connection
- A sense of calm when loved ones are near

These moments become priceless.

What's Happening In The Brain

Stage Seven is the result of widespread, irreversible damage across almost every region of the brain.

Let's break it down in clear terms.

1. The Cerebral Cortex Is Severely Affected

The cortex controls:
- Thinking
- Speaking
- Understanding
- Initiating movement
- Personality
- Awareness

As it deteriorates, these abilities fade significantly.

2. Motor Areas Decline

This primarily affects:

- Walking
- Sitting
- Swallowing
- Hand movements
- Coordination

Neurons cannot carry instructions to muscles effectively, resulting in stiffness, rigidity, or limpness.

3. The Language Centers Are Nearly Silent

Speech becomes:

- Incoherent
- One or two words at a time
- Or disappears completely

People may still understand tone and emotion even when they cannot understand words.

4. The Body's Automatic Functions Struggle

The brainstem and related structures regulate:

- Swallow reflex
- Cough reflex
- Sleep cycles
- Breathing patterns

As these decline, risks increase, including aspiration pneumonia.

5. Emotional Memory Still Exists

Even when other cognitive functions are gone, the brain still responds to:

- Music
- Soothing voices
- Touch
- Familiar scents
- Prayer
- Lullabies
- Soft light

This is because emotional memory is stored in deeper brain structures that are affected later in the disease.

In plain language: Even when a person cannot speak, walk, or swallow, **they can still feel love.**

The Person's Inner Experience

We often ask ourselves:

- "What is their inner world like now?"
- "What do they understand?"
- "Are they scared?"
- "Do they know we're here?"

While every person is different, research and experience show that:

- They may not understand words, but they understand tone.
- They may not recognize faces, but they recognize presence.
- They may not recall names, but they feel safety.
- They may not remember moments, but they feel comfort.
- They may not speak, but they respond emotionally.
- A gentle voice, a soft touch, or a familiar song can calm fear and bring peace.

Their inner world is not empty, it is simply quieter, more fragile, more instinctive.

They live in a place where comfort outweighs understanding, where sensory impressions matter more than memory, and where peace becomes the greatest gift that you can offer.

Daily Life In Stage Seven

Daily life now revolves around:

- Comfort
- Safety
- Dignity
- Tenderness
- Presence

Let's look at the major areas of care.

1. Mobility Declines Sharply

The person may first require:

- Assistance walking
- Then a wheelchair
- Then total support to sit
- Eventually, they become bedridden

This is due to:

- Muscle rigidity
- Brain-body communication breakdown
- Loss of coordination
- Fatigue

Caregiver strategies:

- Use gentle range-of-motion exercises
- Reposition regularly to prevent bedsores
- Use soft bedding
- Ensure proper support for limbs and neck
- Use lifts or transfer devices (to prevent injury)

2. Speech Fades Away

Communication becomes limited to:

- One or two words
- Repetitive phrases
- Moans or sounds
- Facial expressions
- Eye contact
- Hand squeezes
- Eventually, words may disappear entirely.

Caregiver strategies:

- Talk to them anyway
- Use short, simple sentences
- Maintain eye contact
- Use expressive tone
- Pay attention to nonverbal cues

Even silence can be a form of connection.

3. Eating and Swallowing Become Difficult

Dysphagia (difficulty swallowing) is common.

The person may:

- Hold food in their mouth
- Pocket food in their cheeks
- Cough or choke
- Lose weight
- Refuse food
- Sleep through meals

Caregiver strategies:

- Offer soft foods or purees
- Provide small bites
- Allow extra time
- Sit upright to reduce aspiration risk
- Consult hospice or speech therapy for swallowing techniques

In late Stage Seven, the body naturally begins reducing the need for food.

4. Total Incontinence

This is due to:

- Muscle weakness
- Reduced brain signaling
- Loss of awareness
- Immobility

Caregiver strategies:

- Use protective garments
- Keep skin clean and dry
- Apply barrier creams
- Change positions often
- Maintain gentle dignity

5. Sleep Becomes More Frequent

The person may:

- Sleep 18–20 hours a day
- Drift in and out of awareness
- Appear unresponsive at times

This is not giving up, it is a natural part of the body slowing down and ultimately shutting down.

6. Awareness Fades, But Emotion Remains

The person may not:

- Recognize loved ones
- Understand surroundings
- Know their location
- Remember their past

But they can still:

- Feel comfort
- Sense love
- Experience peace
- Respond to familiar stimuli
- Relax in your presence
- Connection becomes energetic, not cognitive.

A Story From this Stage

My mother, Betty, had always been the definition of a social butterfly. She loved people. She loved conversation. She loved laughing, teasing, sharing stories, and making others feel seen. When our videos began going viral on social media, millions of strangers fell in love with her zippy humor, her quick remarks, her warmth. Talking was her superpower.

But as dementia progressed and slipped into its later stages, that superpower slowly quieted.

Our conversations changed.

The long, chatty back-and-forths became shorter.

Her responses became slower.

Her words came only with gentle prompting.

I would ask her simple questions:

"How are you doing today, Mom?"

"What did you have for breakfast?"

"What are we making for dinner?"

But toward the end, I wasn't really asking for information. I was leading her through familiar patterns, like walking hand-in-hand through sentences she could no longer complete on her own.

She would search for a word, her eyes wandering upward as if the right syllable might be hiding on the ceiling. I could see the struggle, the pause, the moment of panic when her mind couldn't connect the dots.

And because I was so in tune with her, because after all these years I knew the rhythms of her thoughts, I could finish her sentences, or give her the missing word. And as soon as I did, she would brighten. She would smile. She would relax, relieved that once again she didn't have to carry the burden alone.

My father and I had become her security blanket, her voice when words failed, her advocates when confusion clouded her world, her translators when her mind could no longer express what her heart still felt. She trusted us to help her communicate, and we did. We always did. It was one of the final gifts we could give her.

But nothing prepared me for that last week.

The week she died is etched into me like a scar I wear with both pain and tenderness. Mom had eaten almost nothing for days. We blended food, tried to coax her with eye droppers of nourishment, but her body had already begun the slow, sacred shutting down that comes at the end of life. She slept more. She drifted in and out of awareness. Her strength was gone. Her words were nearly gone.

At this point, we had a full-time caregiver who typically left around five each evening. The routine was always the same: she would help change Mom, get her settled in bed, and I would come downstairs to be part of the nightly ritual, to assist, to whisper goodnight, to tuck her in with the familiarity she found comforting.

But that Wednesday, just two days before she died, something shifted.

Maybe they started a little early.

Maybe I was distracted with work.

Maybe time slipped faster than usual.

Whatever the reason, by the time I came downstairs, the caregiver was on her way out the door and Mom was already tucked into bed.

I headed straight to her room.

When I entered, she was awake, more awake than she had been all week. Her eyes were open. She was looking right at me. She smiled the moment I sat beside her bed.

I took her hand.

I looked into her eyes.

And I talked to her.

Her responses came out as soft babbling, sounds rather than words, syllables instead of sentences. None of it made sense linguistically, but emotionally? It was perfect. It was her voice. Her effort. Her spirit.

So, I responded as if I understood every syllable.

"Yes? Really? Tell me more!"

"You did? That's wonderful!"

"I know, Mom. I know."

Each time I answered, her face lit up. She smiled wider. She babbled more, her tone rising and falling in the exact musical cadence she'd used when she still had words. And somehow, without comprehension, without vocabulary, we had one of the best conversations of our entire lives.

Fifteen minutes of pure connection.

Fifteen minutes of shared presence.

Fifteen minutes of love spoken without a single recognizable word.

It wasn't conversation as the world defines it.

It was conversation as love defines it.

Two days later, she was gone.

In the days after her passing, that moment replayed in my heart over and over again. Amid the shock and the grief and the quiet house, that memory glowed like a candle; soft, warm, steady.

I was so grateful I came downstairs.

So grateful I didn't miss it.

So grateful she wasn't alone.

So grateful I listened, not to her words, but to her heart.

In those final moments, she didn't have memory.

She didn't have language.

But she had feeling.

And she knew, without question, that she was loved.

I believe with everything in me that she may not have remembered what we talked about... **but she remembered how I made her feel.**

And in Stage Seven, that is everything.

Stage Seven is where dementia strips away almost everything the world uses to define a person: words, movement, appetite, energy, recognition, independence. It is the stage where the body grows quiet and the mind grows distant. It is the stage families dread and the stage caregivers brace themselves for, yet nothing truly prepares you for it.

But Stage Seven also reveals something sacred:
- Even when memory is gone, love is not.
- Even when words disappear, connection remains.
- Even when the mind is fading, the heart still knows.

What happened that Wednesday night was more than a sweet moment. It was the essence of Stage Seven itself, a reminder that communication is deeper than language, and presence is more powerful than memory.

In this final stage:

You don't love through conversation.

You love through tone.

Through touch.

Through patience.

Through stillness.

Through staying.

You love by showing up, even when they cannot.

You love by listening to what can't be spoken.

You love by offering peace to a mind that no longer knows how to ask for it.

This is the stage where caregivers learn the truth:

The most meaningful conversations at the end of life rarely involve words.

They involve presence.

That last "conversation" with my mother, fifteen minutes of babbling and smiles, was not a medical milestone. It was a spiritual one. A soul-level one. It was her last gift to me and my last sacred moment with her.

And it reminded me that Stage Seven, though heartbreaking, is also holy.

It is the stage where love becomes its purest form; wordless, boundless, unconditional, and eternal.

The Role Of Caregivers In Stage Seven

Caregivers now become:

- Comfort-givers
- Gentle attendants
- Advocates
- Protectors
- Companions
- Sacred witnesses

The goal shifts from independence to comfort.

From support to soothing.

From activity to presence.

From prolonging life to preserving peace.

Caregivers may experience:

- Deep grief
- Exhaustion
- Tenderness
- Sacred connection
- Heartbreak
- Guilt

- Spiritual reflection
- Anticipatory grief

This is one of the hardest stages, and one of the holiest.

What Helps Most In Stage Seven

Soft music:

- Music accesses deep emotional memory.

Gentle touch:

- Hand-holding
- Brushing hair
- Rubbing shoulders
- Applying lotion

These communicate safety.

Calm voice:

- Even if they don't understand the words.

Familiar scents:

- Lotions, perfumes, or household smells can soothe.

Prayer or scripture:

- If the person has faith, it can bring peace.

Environment:

- Soft lighting, quiet rooms, comfortable bedding.

Hospice support which offers:

- Pain management
- Skilled nursing
- Emotional support
- Guidance for families

Hospice does not mean giving or a death sentence.

It means embracing comfort.

The Final Days And Hours

In the final stage of dementia, the body naturally begins shutting down. Common signs include:

- Long pauses in breathing
- Cool hands or feet
- Sleeping with eyes partially open
- Minimal response to touch
- Decreased appetite and thirst
- Peaceful stillness

- Restlessness
- Facial muscles relaxing
- Shallow breaths

Caregivers often say the room feels "holy."

A quietness settles in.

Time slows.

Your presence is the greatest gift:
- Sitting beside them
- Holding their hand
- Speaking softly
- Being there without needing anything in return

Death in dementia is not the person "giving up."

It is the natural conclusion of a long journey.

Many caregivers say they feel their loved one slipping peacefully, gently, like a candle flickering out.

What Remains After Memory Is Gone

This stage teaches us the deepest truth of dementia:

Memory is not required for love.

Cognition is not required for connection.

Awareness is not required for dignity.

When everything else falls away, love remains:
- Love through presence
- Love through touch
- Love through silence
- Love through patience
- Love through tears
- Love through goodbye

Stage Seven is the place where love becomes unconditional, where it becomes an act of devotion rather than dialogue.

Grief And The Caregiver

Caregivers in Stage Seven grieve on multiple levels:
- The loss of the person they used to know
- The loss of shared conversation
- The loss of mobility and expression
- The loss of recognition
- The loss of daily routines together
- The anticipation of death
- The exhaustion of long-term caregiving
- The sacred intimacy of the final days

But they also discover:
- the strength of their love
- the depth of their patience

- the resilience of their spirit
- the meaning in small gestures
- the beauty of presence
- the holiness of caring for someone at life's end

The End Of The Journey

When the final moment comes, it is often:

- Peaceful
- Quiet
- Gentle
- Sacred

As the body relaxes, breathing slows, and the final breath arrives, many caregivers hold their loved one's hand and whisper:

"It's okay. You can rest now. I love you."

And in that moment, something extraordinary happens:

Grief and gratitude meet for the first time.

Grief, because the journey has ended.

Gratitude, because you were there for every step of it.

The Legacy Of Stage Seven

Stage Seven leaves behind:

- A legacy of courage
- A legacy of love
- A legacy of devotion
- A legacy of forgiveness
- A legacy of presence

No person is defined by dementia.

Not by forgetting.

Not by confusion.

Not by physical decline.

Not by the final stage.

They are defined by:

- the life they lived
- the love they gave
- the memories they created
- and the hearts they touched

Stage Seven is not the end of the story, it's **walking them home.**

THINGS I LEARNED
ALONG MY JOURNEY

"If I'm honest, I didn't know I was becoming a caregiver until the job had already broken me."

If someone had told me years ago that I would one day write a book about Alzheimer's disease... about caregiving... about grief and decline and dignity and love... I wouldn't have believed them. Not because I didn't love my mother enough to tell her story, but because I never imagined that this disease would choose our family. I never imagined it would choose her.

My mother, Betty, was one of the sharpest, most vibrant, most socially alive people you could ever meet. She was a woman who remembered everything; every birthday, every recipe, every detail of every story she told. She ran organizations, traveled the country, lifted spirits everywhere she went, and held our family together with the kind of effortless strength you don't appreciate until life tests it.

Alzheimer's tested it.
Alzheimer's tested *all* of us.

But nothing prepares you for the slow, painful shift from "child" to "caregiver."
No class teaches you how to watch your mother's mind fade.
No doctor prepares you for how quickly roles reverse.
No pamphlet explains the heartbreak of losing someone who is still alive.

Caregiving doesn't arrive all at once. It seeps in quietly, through moments that feel small at first:

A repeated question.
A misplaced object.
A forgotten step in a familiar routine.
A look of confusion where there used to be certainty.

And before you know it...you've become the navigator of someone else's disappearing world.

I didn't recognize the signs in the beginning.
I didn't understand the progression.
I didn't know the emotional toll it would take.
I didn't know how heavy it would be... until I was carrying all of it.

This book is not a medical textbook. It's not a clinical guide. It's not written by a professional with decades of letters behind their name. It's written by a son.

A son who loved his mother so deeply that he fought this disease with every ounce of compassion he could find.

A son who learned the hard way, through **mistakes**, through **breakdowns**, through **sleepless nights** and **desperate prayers**, how to care for someone with Alzheimer's. A son who walked this journey with his father, watching how love can stretch and break and rebuild itself again during the hardest years of life. A son who held his mother's hand as she slipped further and further away... and who still believes that even in the decline, there is beauty worth sharing.

The chapters ahead are seven truths that carved themselves into me during the eleven years I cared for my mother, truths I wish someone had handed to me at the start of this journey. Truths I now hand to you.

If you are caring for someone with Alzheimer's...
If you love someone who is disappearing a little more every day...
If you feel alone, overwhelmed, guilty, angry, exhausted, or broken...

You are not failing.
You are not weak.
You are not alone.

This book is for you. To sit with you. To steady you. To tell you the truth with gentleness and honesty. To show you that what you feel is normal, and survivable. To remind you that love is still happening, even when memory is not. And most importantly...

To walk with you through **the seven hardest, most transformative lessons I learned** while caregiving: lessons that reshaped my heart, my patience, my understanding, and my life.

LESSON 1:
THE UNAVOIDABLE TRUTH: THINGS WILL ALWAYS GET WORSE

"You cannot fight a disease that only moves forward, but you can choose how you walk beside it."

One of the hardest lessons in Alzheimer's caregiving is also the one nobody wants to say out loud: **things will get worse.**

Not because you aren't doing enough.

Not because you're failing.

Not because of treatment choices or effort or attitude or prayer.

But because Alzheimer's only moves in one direction, and that direction is away from the person you once knew.

I resisted this truth for a long time and clung to denial like it was life support.

I held onto hope in a way that wasn't really hope. Part of that denial came from who my mother had always been.

Betty was *sharp*. She was witty. She could tell you the birthdate of a cousin she hadn't seen in twenty years, the ingredients of a recipe she hadn't made since I was a kid, or a story from forty years ago with crystal clarity. She was a woman of details… precise ones.

So when the earliest signs of decline crept in, we did what most families do: we explained them away.

"She's tired."

"She's stressed."

"She's getting older."

"It's just normal aging."

We didn't know that Alzheimer's rarely announces itself. It whispers first. And when you don't yet understand the language of the disease, those whispers go unnoticed.

By the time the neurologist said the words *moderate to severe Alzheimer's disease*, Mom was already in Stage Five.

We didn't know it. We didn't see it. We were too distracted by her cancer diagnoses, the surgeries, the treatments, the constant medical appointments. Cancer was loud. Dementia was quiet. And in those quiet spaces, it grew.

The Day Hope Became Denial

When we first received the Alzheimer's diagnosis, the doctor prescribed Donepezil. I remember feeling a strange wave of relief wash over me.

A medication.

A plan.

Something we could do.

We were conditioned by every other illness we had ever faced, to believe that treatment leads to improvement.

But Alzheimer's doesn't play by those rules.

We gave the medication time. We wanted to believe. But the questions kept repeating.

The skin picking got worse. The memory gaps widened. The confusion deepened.

We returned to the neurologist, frustrated and certain the medication he had given us wasn't working. We were certain something had been missed or that we needed to try something else.

That's when he said something that changed the entire trajectory of my caregiving journey.

"She's not going to get better."

His voice wasn't cold, it was compassionate, but firm.

"You're treating this disease like you treat her cancer," he continued. "You're expecting a response. Improvement. Stabilization. But Alzheimer's only moves one way. These medications might *slow* the progression, but they will not reverse it."

He paused, letting the truth settle in the room like smoke.

"You're getting frustrated because she can't remember what you told her ten minutes ago. But she *has dementia*. She *cannot* remember. The problem isn't her. The problem is that you expect her to act like she doesn't have the disease."

His words were a punch to the gut.

A necessary, painful punch.

That was the day I learned the first great truth of caregiving:

You cannot help someone with Alzheimer's if you are still holding onto who they used to be.

Decline Does Not Mean Failure

Once I accepted that this disease only moves in one direction, something shifted inside me, slowly at first, then completely.

I stopped evaluating her days through the lens of "better or worse."

I stopped clinging to the version of her from the year before.

I stopped expecting improvement.

And in that acceptance, harsh as it was, I found a strange, unexpected relief.

Not relief that she was declining.

Relief that I could stop fighting what was already happening.

Relief that I could stop blaming myself when she slipped further.

Relief that I could meet her where she was instead of dragging her toward where I wished she still could be.

Decline is not failure.

Decline is the nature of Alzheimer's.

Once you know that, you stop interpreting every symptom as a crisis, and you start interpreting them as part of the journey.

The Day She Forgot How To Get Into the Car

There was a moment, small to an outsider, devastating to me, when I realized decline was happening faster than my denial could keep up with.

I was helping Mom into the car. Something she had done tens of thousands of times in her life.

But this time, she froze.

She stared at the open door like she had never seen a car interior before.

She couldn't figure out where to put her hands. She couldn't remember whether to lead with her left foot or her right. She could not compute the physical sequence.

Her eyes searched mine, not for help, but for permission to not know what to do.

That broke me.

Not because she was declining, but because she *knew* she was declining.

The confusion wasn't just inside her brain.

It was written all over her face.

And I realized that every moment I expected her to act like her old self was a moment I unintentionally added pressure to a mind already fighting for its life.

The Invisible Grief of Decline
Alzheimer's forces you into a long, slow grief, one that begins long before death and continues through every forgotten memory, every lost ability, every shift in personality.

It is the grief of watching someone fade.

The grief of losing pieces of them in real time.

The grief of saying goodbye over and over without closure.

But it is also the grief of expectations.

You grieve the version of caregiving you thought you'd be doing.

You grieve the mother you remember from childhood.

You grieve the belief that you could somehow protect her from decline.

And you grieve the illusion that you could stop the disease by loving her hard enough.

Accepting decline doesn't stop the grief.
It simply makes space for compassion.

The Raw Lesson Every Caregiver Must Learn
This is the truth I wish someone had handed me on day one:

Alzheimer's is a disease of continual loss, but when you stop expecting things to get better, you finally become free to love the person in front of you as they are today.

Not as they were yesterday.

Not as you wish they could be.

But as they are right now, in this moment, in this stage, with these abilities, and this version of themselves.

You stop teaching.

You stop correcting.

You stop resisting.

You stop waiting for improvement that will never come.

And you start *loving* without *expectation*.

That is the first, hardest, most liberating step of caregiving.

LESSON 2:
THE RHYTHM OF PEACE: WHY ROUTINE MATTERS MORE THAN YOU THINK

"Looking back, I realize it wasn't the hard days that broke her, it was the days I rushed her, pushed her, or pulled her out of the rhythm her brain depended on."

If the last chapter teaches you that Alzheimer's always moves forward, this chapter teaches you something equally important:

A predictable world is a peaceful world for someone with dementia.

Alzheimer's strips away memory, reasoning, sequencing, and the ability to navigate change. Routine becomes the scaffolding that holds up the pieces of their shrinking world. And the moment that scaffolding wobbles, everything else does too.

I didn't understand this at first.

My life was built on spontaneity, flexible work hours, unpredictable days, lots of "we'll just figure it out." I could start work at a coffee shop one day and in my home office the next. I'd say, "Let's go here," or "Let's run errands now," and never think twice about how last-minute changes would feel to someone whose mind was already overwhelmed.

To me, the day was fluid.

To her, the day needed anchors.

And once I understood that, everything changed.

A Brain Without Short-Term Memory Live In Constant Uncertainty

For someone with Alzheimer's, routine is more than habit, it's orientation. It's safety. It's the last thing their brain can rely on.

Imagine waking up each morning in a world where nothing feels familiar, not the time, not the day, not what's coming next, not what's expected of you.

Imagine knowing that something is wrong in your mind but not knowing *what* or *why*. Imagine the fear of feeling lost inside your own life.

Now imagine the relief when one thing stays the same:

- Breakfast always happens at the same time.
- The shower always comes after breakfast.
- Your walk always happens after lunch.
- Your son always sits beside you in the afternoons.
- Dinner always happens before the nighttime routine.

Predictability isn't boring for someone with dementia. Predictability is freedom.

Because when the next step is always the same, they don't have to rely on the part of the brain that is failing.

Routine becomes memory's substitute.

And once I learned that, I stopped trying to fit my mother into *my* schedule and began shaping our lives around *hers*.

The Day I Learned Routine Wasn't Optional

My lightbulb moment came in the fall of 2023, when The Charlotte Observer came to interview us during the height of Mom's second wave of viral fame. The reporter and photographer were scheduled to arrive in the early afternoon.

Our normal routine at that time was simple: A caregiver came a few days a week. She would help give Mom a shower after lunch, but only after Dad and I had left the house. Mom handled showering better when we weren't there. With us, she resisted. With the caregiver alone, it became "getting ready before they get home," and she cooperated beautifully.

But that day, we decided to shift everything.

We wanted Mom to look nice for the interview, so we brought the caregiver in early and tried to squeeze the shower in before the reporters arrived.

It sounded reasonable. Logical, even.

Except to Mom's brain, it was chaos.

We rushed her breakfast. We hovered in the bathroom trying to assist the caregiver with the shower. We pushed her into a task that usually went smoothly only when done the same way it always was. Dad and I were yelling instructions, trying to make her cooperate.

And everything fell apart.

She became agitated, confused, and stubborn, the kind of stubborn that comes from fear, not defiance.

The routine was broken, the sequencing shattered, and she couldn't find her footing.

Then came the moment that still stings when I replay it.

In the middle of all the pressure and coaxing, Mom went limp, not a fall, but the passive collapse that people with advanced dementia sometimes do when overwhelmed. She gently lowered herself to the floor, unable to process the next instruction.

And suddenly our mission to "make her look nice" felt cruel, misguided and selfish.

She didn't need to be beautiful for the media. She needed to feel safe. Routine was her safety. And I had bulldozed right through it.

Routine Isn't About Control, It's About Reducing Fear

After that day, it became painfully clear:

- Every time we broke her routine, her behavior changed.
- Her anxiety spiked.
- Her confusion deepened.
- Her cooperation vanished.

But when we leaned into the rhythm her mind depended on, she was calmer. She laughed more. She trusted us more. She had fewer meltdowns and almost no resistance to daily tasks.

Routine is not about forcing structure. It is about giving the brain a shortcut.

A familiar sequence bypasses the damaged parts of memory and creates a sense of flow:
- "This comes after that."
- "Breakfast means the caregiver will be here soon."
- "Lunch means we are getting ready for a walk."
- "Evening means bedtime is safe and predictable."

When you remove surprise, you remove fear. When you remove fear, you remove resistance. When you remove resistance, caregiving becomes peaceful instead of combative.

Learning this truth changed everything about how I approached my mother's day.

The Smallest Disruptions Cause the Biggest Reactions
One of the things Alzheimer's teaches you, painfully, is that the size of the disruption does not match the size of the reaction.

A small change can feel catastrophic to their brain.

A different order of the day.

A rushed meal.

A new caregiver.

A sudden outing.

A change in the lighting, noise level, or environment.

A skipped step in the routine.

While you or I may see these things as minor, to someone whose world is already slipping away, these can feel like earthquakes.

But here's the beautiful part:

Consistency gives them back a sense of control, even if they cannot communicate that.

The Beauty Of Letting the Day Unfold Their Way
Once we embraced Mom's routine, truly embraced it, the entire house shifted.

Meals happened at the same times. Showers were never rushed. Caregiver days followed the same flow every week. Outings were planned around her best hours. Visitors were timed with predictability in mind. New tasks were introduced slowly and gently.

There were fewer accidents. Fewer meltdowns. Fewer moments of panic. Fewer heartbreaking expressions of being overwhelmed.

In honoring her rhythm, we found ours.

And in that rhythm, caregiving became less of a struggle and more of a partnership.

The Raw Lesson Every Caregiver Must Learn
This chapter boils down to one truth:

Your routine may be flexible, but their routine cannot be.

When you honor the rhythm their brain depends on, everything becomes gentler:
- They resist less.
- They trust more.
- They feel safer.
- They move through the day with more confidence.

And you, as the caregiver, stop fighting battles that never needed to happen.

Routine doesn't cure Alzheimer's. But it stabilizes the emotional ground beneath it.

It is one of the greatest gifts you can give someone whose mind is slipping:

A world that stays the same.

A sequence they can count on.

A rhythm that makes their life feel safe again.

LESSON 3:
IT'S NOT THEM. IT'S THE DISEASE.

"The day I stopped taking her behavior personally was the day I finally saw my mother again, beneath the disease that was stealing her from me."

There is a moment in every caregiver's journey when the frustration becomes unbearable.

A moment when the behaviors, the refusals, the repeating questions, the agitation, the irrational arguments reach a point where your patience feels like it's hanging by a thread.

I reached that moment many times.

Not because I didn't love my mother.

Not because I wasn't trying hard enough.

But because I was human.

And caregiving pushes every emotional boundary a person has.

But something changed the day I finally understood a truth that would reshape the way I showed up for my mom, a truth I wish I had embraced much sooner:

It's not them. It's the disease.

Those six words freed me.

They softened me.

They helped me see her clearly again.

Because Alzheimer's is not just memory loss.

- It is personality loss.
- Reasoning loss.
- Emotional regulation loss.
- Inhibition loss.
- Judgment loss.
- Self-control loss.
- Sequencing loss.
- Reality loss.

And when you don't understand those losses, you will interpret their behavior as intentional. But once you do understand, everything changes.

When Alzheimer's Steals the Filters

My mother, Betty, was one of the sweetest, most gentle, most kindhearted people you could meet. She poured love into everyone, her family, her church, her community, her friends. She had grace for everyone.

But Alzheimer's stripped away her filters.

The disease removed her ability to self-regulate.

It took away the part of her brain that said:
- "This is appropriate."
- "This is kind."
- "This is logical."
- "This is safe."

And when that happens, you see behaviors that don't match the person you remember:
- Agitation.
- Irritability.
- Suspicion.
- Stubbornness.
- Paranoia.
- Fear.
- Anger.
- Confusion.

At first, I interpreted all of that as "Mom being difficult."

I took it personally. I argued. I corrected. I insisted. I tried to reason.

And every time I did, I thought I was helping.

I wasn't. I was escalating her fear.

Because behind every "stubborn moment" was not a stubborn woman, but a frightened brain trying to make sense of a world that no longer made sense.

The Day Dina Gave Me the Sentence That Saved My Sanity

We were blessed to have an extraordinary caregiver, Dina. She had known my parents long before Alzheimer's entered our world, and she had seen the change with compassionate eyes.

One day, Mom was resisting something simple, eating, or walking, or going to the bathroom, I don't even remember the task anymore. What I remember is my frustration.

I was trying everything, coaxing, explaining, yelling, negotiating.

I was losing patience.

She was losing trust.

And that's when Dina gently stepped beside me, placed her hand on my shoulder, and said the sentence that would change the rest of my caregiving journey:

"Josh... it's not her. It's the disease."

The words hit me like a wave.

I stopped. I exhaled. Something in me surrendered.

Dina knew my mother before she was sick, so she knew how my mother would and would not have acted. But she also knew this disease could make people act differently. I was too close to see it.

She wasn't choosing this behavior.

She wasn't trying to frustrate me.

She wasn't being difficult.

She wasn't disagreeing on purpose.

She wasn't refusing because she wanted control.

Her brain was failing her. Her disease was speaking louder than her personality. And once that clicked, my entire perspective shifted.

The Real Betty vs. The Disease

One of the most powerful exercises I began practicing was this:

Each time Mom reacted in a way that didn't make sense, I asked myself this question.

"Is this Betty… or is this Alzheimer's?"

And almost every time, the answer was Alzheimer's.

The real Betty would never:
- Resist help out of stubbornness
- Lash out suddenly
- Cry without understanding why
- Accuse someone of something that wasn't true
- Forget a face she loved
- Repeat the same question every ten minutes

The real Betty was still there, but the disease was speaking over her.

When I separated the two, I could love her again without resentment, frustration or blame.

It felt like peeling back the fog to find her heart again.

The Story Of the Bingo Table

Before Alzheimer's, Mom ran the household finances. She balanced checkbooks. She kept track of bills, receipts, records, all of it.

So when she and Dad volunteered at bingo in their retirement community, she naturally handled the money selling boards. These were small dollar transactions, $1 per board, nothing complicated. But Dad began noticing something was off.

She hesitated with making change. She second-guessed herself. She would hand him the money and say, "Check me."

It wasn't a math problem. It was a sequencing problem... a cognitive processing issue which was a symptom of the disease.

At the time, Dad chalked it up to aging. We all did.

But looking back, that was Alzheimer's whispering its earliest warnings.

Not incompetence. Not carelessness. Not irresponsibility.

It was the disease.

And once I reframed it as the disease, I stopped feeling the disappointment I once felt. I stopped seeing the moments as failures. I started seeing them as signals — signs that she needed patience, not correction.

The Moment Eye Contact Disappeared

Dad once told me the first sign that scared him was when Mom stopped making eye contact with others in conversations.

She had always looked people right in the eye.

She was present, fully present.

But then, slowly, she started looking down or looking away and looking at Dad for reassurance, as if checking whether her story made sense, whether her details were correct, whether she was saying the right thing.

That wasn't insecurity.

That wasn't disinterest.

That wasn't rudeness.

It was the disease interfering with the part of the brain that handles social cues. Her brain was losing its ability to follow the thread of conversation, the sequencing, the memory, the context.

Her eyes were scanning for help.

Once you realize that, you never again misinterpret the withdrawn gaze of a person with dementia.

You see the fear behind it.

You see the effort.

You see the exhaustion.

You see the person trying desperately to stay connected even as the disease pulls them away.

The Emotional Reframe That Changes Everything
The moment you understand that the behavior is the disease, not the person, something sacred happens in your caregiving relationship:

Compassion returns. Patience expands.

The guilt from your frustration softens. The resentment dissolves. The anger evaporates. Your heart opens again.

You can finally stop arguing. Stop correcting. Stop demanding logic. Stop expecting them to be the person they were before.

Instead, you begin responding from empathy, not irritation.

Because once you see the disease as the source of the behavior, you stop fighting the person and start fighting for them.

Alzheimer's Is a Thief, Not A Choice
This disease steals:
- Memory
- Mobility
- Language
- Identity
- Logic
- Patience
- Self-regulation
- Confidence
- Dignity
- Time

And if you're not careful, it can steal your relationship, too.

But it doesn't have to.

When you separate the disease from the person...

You begin to grieve the symptoms without blaming the one who has them.

You begin to see the fear behind the confusion.

You begin to protect their dignity instead of their accuracy.

You begin to respond with gentleness instead of frustration.

You begin to love them with a deeper, truer love, a love unclouded by expectation.

The Raw Lesson Every Caregiver Must Learn
Here is the truth that defines this chapter:

Your loved one is not giving you a hard time. Your loved one *is having* a hard time.

And once you believe that, truly believe it, you will stop taking things personally.

You will stop arguing logic with a disease that cannot understand logic.

You will stop expecting consistency from a brain that can no longer deliver it.

You will stop measuring their intentions by their behavior.

Your heart will break a hundred times on this journey. But it will also soften in ways you never knew it could. And at the end of it, when the disease has taken everything it can take, you will know that you loved the person, not the symptoms.

LESSON 4:
LIVE IN THEIR WORLD

"The moment I stopped dragging her into my world and instead stepped into hers, everything softened... her fears, her resistance, and my frustration."

If there is one lesson that would have saved me years of stress, arguments, tears, and exhaustion, it is this one:

You cannot bring a person with Alzheimer's into your world. You must join them in theirs.

I didn't understand this in the beginning.
Honestly, I didn't even understand it in the middle.
It took me far too long to realize that logic, truth, and correction were anchors, anchors I kept throwing at my mother, thinking they would steady her, when in reality they only pulled her deeper into confusion.

Because here's the truth about dementia:

Their reality is not wrong. It is simply different.

And no amount of arguing will pull them out of it.
But love, gentle, flexible, compassionate love, can walk beside them inside it.

Why Arguing with Alzheimer's Never Works

The neurologist once told us:

"Expecting someone with dementia to learn something new is the definition of insanity."

At the time, it felt like he was exaggerating. He wasn't.

A person with Alzheimer's cannot:
- Retain new information
- Reason through explanations
- Break habits through logic
- Be corrected into reality
- Remember what you just clarified

And yet, that is exactly what most caregivers try to do in the beginning.

We debate. We correct. We explain. We remind. We insist. We argue.

Why?

Because we want to anchor them in truth. Because we want to pull them out of confusion. Because we think if we repeat things enough times, they'll stick.

They won't.

Alzheimer's erases new information faster than you can speak it.

So every attempt to correct them becomes another wound, for them and for you.

The moment you realize this, the moment you stop trying to force them into your world...
peace enters the room.

The Sky Is Green
"Yes, and it's beautiful today."

I always tell new caregivers this simple rule:

If they say the sky is green, tell them it's the prettiest shade you've ever seen.

Not because you're choosing to lie.

Not because you're giving up truth.

But because you're choosing connection over correction.

People with dementia aren't trying to deceive you.

They are telling you what they believe, based on the information their brain is giving them.

Correcting them only introduces distress.

Agreeing with them introduces peace.

When Keeping the Peace Matters More Than Keeping the Facts

When Mom began slipping deeper into the disease, she often entered her own time periods, her childhood, her early marriage years, moments from decades ago.

Sometimes she believed her father was alive. Sometimes she thought her brother was still around. Sometimes she wondered when her parents were visiting.

In the early days, we corrected her.

"No Mom, your father passed years ago."

"No, your brother died."

"No, that person isn't alive anymore."

We thought we were helping. We thought she deserved the truth.

But every time we told her, she grieved them **again**. Every single time.

Imagine reliving a death you've already mourned... every day, sometimes several times a day.

We realized very quickly:

Telling the truth can be cruel when the truth cannot be retained.

So we stopped.

If she asked about her father, we said: "He's not here right now, but he's doing okay."

If she asked about her brother, we said: "He's safe. Don't worry about him."

Those statements were not lies. They were bridges, bridges that allowed her to stay calm, stay comforted, stay connected.

This disease steals so much. There is no need to let it steal peace too.

Living In Their World Doesn't Mean Giving Up
It Means Showing Up.

Stepping into their reality is not surrender, it is love, pure, unconditional love.

It means saying:
- "I choose your comfort over my need to be right."
- "I choose connection over accuracy."
- "I choose compassion over explanation."

- "I choose your world over the one you can no longer stay in."

It means stopping the arguments before they begin.

It means softening instead of correcting.

It means seeing the person, not the confusion.

The Gift of Lexi: A Lesson in Gentle Redirection
Sometimes living in their world means becoming a creative partner in their reality.

We had a family friend, Lexi, who would sit with Mom occasionally while Dad and I went to church golf group. She was a natural, calm, warm, intuitive.

One night, Mom became anxious, worried about when we were coming home.

Where were we?

Why weren't we back yet?

Had something happened?

Had we forgotten her?
Her confusion was growing into fear.

Lexi didn't correct her. She didn't argue or explain. She didn't scold or lecture.

She simply said, "Oh, they just texted me, they're on their way. They should be here soon."

And then, with a little mischievous smile, she added: "They're probably taking so long because they're terrible golfers."

Mom laughed. And since mom found the most humor poking fun at my father, every time Lexi repeated it, she laughed again.

Ten minutes later, when she asked the same question, Lexi used the exact same script.

And it worked. Every single time.

Because Mom didn't need the truth. She needed reassurance. She needed familiarity. She needed comfort.

She needed someone to live in the moment with her, not drag her into a reality she could no longer hold onto.

The Freedom of Letting Go of Reality
It may sound strange, but when I finally let go of forcing Mom into the real world, I felt something I hadn't felt in years:

Relief.

I didn't have to correct her. I didn't have to fix her understanding. I didn't have to argue. I didn't have to force clarity into a brain that could no longer hold clarity.

All I had to do was love her.

And suddenly, our connection grew stronger. Our days felt easier. Her fear decreased. Her trust increased. Our home became calmer.

Because when you stop battling reality, the disease no longer feels like an enemy you're wrestling, it becomes a landscape you're navigating together.

The Raw Lesson Every Caregiver Must Learn
This chapter asks you to do something incredibly counterintuitive:

Let go of the world as you know it. Enter the world as they perceive it.

Not because their world is accurate. Not because it makes sense. Not because you enjoy it. But because they are trapped there, and you are not.

You have the ability to cross realities. They do not. So cross. Meet them where they are. Hold their hand in the world they're living in, not the one you wish they could stay in.

Because when you step into their world, something extraordinary happens:

They feel understood.

They feel safe.

They feel loved.

They feel connected.

And even as memory fails... *feelings* remain.

People with dementia may not remember what you said, or what you did, or who visited, or what happened yesterday... but they will remember how you made them feel.

And there is no greater gift you can give them than this:

Peace inside the only world they can still access.

LESSON 5:
THE ART OF DISTRACTION
& REDIRECTION

*"The day I learned that distraction
wasn't manipulation but mercy,
everything about caregiving became gentler...
for her, and for me."*

If there is one skill that separates peaceful caregiving from constant struggle, it is this:

Distraction and redirection.

Not the kind of distraction you use with children. Not the kind of redirection you use to avoid an argument.

But a deeper, more compassionate form, one that honors the limitations of a brain that cannot hold onto a thought, cannot process a sequence, cannot regulate emotion, and cannot reason its way out of fear.

When memory disappears, when logic breaks down, when time loses meaning, when the person you love suddenly looks frightened and doesn't know why... **distraction becomes a lifeline. Redirection becomes a rescue. And together, they become your greatest tools.**

But like everything in dementia caregiving, I didn't understand this at first. And because I didn't understand, I made things harder on all of us, especially on my mother.

Why Distraction Works When Nothing Else Will
When someone with Alzheimer's becomes upset, confused, anxious, or fixated on a thought, their brain cannot reason through it.

You cannot explain them out of their fear. You cannot convince them with facts. You cannot argue them into calmness.

Logic does not soothe a damaged memory center. But a shift of focus can.

Because dementia wipes out short-term memory, a distressing thought may only last seconds, *if* you gently replace it with something new.

This isn't manipulation. It isn't trickery. It's mercy.

It's the art of giving them something more pleasant to hold onto when their mind is gripping something painful.

Once I understood this, truly understood it, my mother's hardest moments became far more manageable.

And my own heart became far less heavy.

The Day I Learned How Powerful Distraction Really Was

One afternoon, I walked downstairs from my office to find Mom sitting at the kitchen counter, sobbing, not quietly, but the deep, broken cry of someone who feels utterly alone in the world.

She wasn't abandoned. She wasn't hurt. She wasn't unsafe. But she didn't know that.

Dad had stepped away for just a moment, to brush his teeth and get ready for the day. But in Mom's perception, he had vanished.

Time no longer meant minutes or hours to her. It became a shapeless, floating void. And in that void, she panicked.

I asked gently, "Mom, what's wrong?"

With tears streaming down her cheeks, she sobbed, "I don't know where Dad is."

Her voice cracked under the weight of fear she could not explain.

I reassured her, "He's just in the bathroom. He'll be right back. He didn't leave you."

But reassurance only went so far. She nodded, but the fear remained.

Then I saw it, a brand-new coffee mug on the counter that a follower had sent. It had her name on it in big, beautiful letters: BETTY.

I picked it up and said, "Mom, look! Did you see your new mug?"

Her tears stopped. Her expression softened. She blinked and leaned closer.

"My mug?" she asked, touching it gently.

Suddenly we were talking about the color, the lettering, the weight of it in her hands.

Within seconds, her sadness was gone.

Not because I solved her problem. Not because I reasoned her out of her fear. But because I gave her mind something else to hold.

In that moment, I realized:

Distraction is not avoidance. It is salvation.

When Redirection Becomes A Love Language
As dementia progresses, many of the things that upset your loved one come from:
- Misinterpretation
- Fear
- Confusion
- Misplaced memories
- Inability to process
- Feeling overwhelmed
- Being stuck on a single thought
- Not recognizing the passage of time

And because their brain cannot untangle those emotions, they get trapped in them.

Distraction is the bridge that carries them out.

Redirection is the hand that guides them across. And love is what makes it work.

Redirection is not dismissing their feelings. It is relieving them of distress their brain can no longer navigate.

It is saying:

"You don't have to carry this thought any longer.
Let me give you something lighter."

How Redirection Saved Us from Countless Meltdowns

There were dozens of moments when distraction and redirection saved us, truly saved us, from spiraling into emotional chaos.

Mom fixated on the same question? → Redirect.

Mom insisted she needed to leave? → Redirect.

Mom believed someone was missing? → Redirect.

Mom refused food? → Redirect with a different plate, different seat, different story.

Mom was scared? → Redirect to something comforting.

Mom was crying? → Redirect to something familiar or joyful.

It was like magic, but not the kind that tricks. The kind that heals.

Because distraction works with the brain as it is, not as we wish it were.

One Of The Most Important Skills You Will Ever Learn
Here is the heart of this chapter:

The moment you see distraction and redirection as compassion instead of deception, caregiving becomes easier, and your loved one becomes calmer.

You are not lying to them. You are relieving them of the emotional weight they cannot put down on their own.

You are not manipulating them. You are giving them a gentle exit from distress.

You are not tricking them. You are protecting them from their own brain.

And as their disease progresses, this skill becomes your lifeline, and their comfort.

Why This Doesn't Work Without Love

You can't redirect with irritation.

You can't distract with frustration.

You can't soothe while you're still angry.

The success of distraction comes from:
- Warm tone
- Soft expression
- Reassuring body language
- Patience
- Consistency
- Meeting them where they are emotionally
- Offering calm energy when theirs is spiraling

A person with dementia may not remember your words, but they will always remember your tone.

If your voice shakes with stress, they will feel it. If your face shows frustration, they will sense it. If your energy is frantic, theirs will escalate.

But if you speak gently, softly, warmly, they will follow your emotional lead.

Distraction works because the heart behind it works.

The Raw Lesson Every Caregiver Must Learn

Here is the essence of this chapter:

Distraction is not avoidance. It is compassion.

Redirection is not deception. It is protection.

These techniques are not tricks. They are acts of mercy, a way to give your loved one peace when their brain is offering them anything but.

Once you see distraction and redirection as tools of love, your days will become gentler,
your stress will decrease, and your connection with your loved one will deepen.

And they will feel safer in your care, because you are guiding them, not correcting them; comforting them, not confronting them; walking with them, not pulling them.

LESSON 6:
LEARN THE SIGNS OF
URINARY TRACT INFECTIONS

"If I could place one warning label on Alzheimer's caregiving, it would be this: sudden changes are not always dementia, sometimes they are danger."

If you've never cared for someone with Alzheimer's or dementia, you might assume that a **urinary tract infection (UTI for short)** is no big deal, something uncomfortable, annoying, easy to treat, and obvious when it happens.

But dementia changes everything.

A UTI in someone with Alzheimer's is not just a UTI. It can be an emotional earthquake. A behavioral explosion. A physical crisis. A sudden and terrifying shift in their cognitive world.

And in the beginning, we didn't know that.

Because UTIs hide inside dementia symptoms so easily, you can mistake them for sudden progression of the disease.

And if you don't know better, you panic, you assume decline, you brace for the worst, you feel helpless.

But once you do know better, you start to see UTIs as what they truly are:

Medical emergencies hiding inside behavioral changes. Treatable crises hidden in plain sight.

And in my experience caring for my mother, learning to recognize UTIs was the difference between fear and control. Between chaos and calm. Between unnecessary suffering and rapid relief.

The Day I Realized Something Was Terribly Wrong
There were many times when UTIs hit my mother without warning, but one in particular is burned into my memory.

She had been doing... okay. Not great, not alert, not her old self, but steady in the familiar way of late-stage Alzheimer's.

While I was sick with the flu and quarantined upstairs, downstairs, dad watched her try to stand from her chair to go get ready for bed, and she couldn't.

Not because she was weak. Not because she was tired. Not because she forgot how. She simply couldn't bear her own weight.

Her eyes looked distant, her body limp, her mind fogged over with a confusion that felt heavier than usual. She could not get up, and my father was unable to help her up.

It wasn't the "normal" dementia fog. It was deeper. Darker. Quicker in its arrival.

And instantly, instinctively, we knew:

Check for a UTI.

Sure enough, that was the cause.

One antibiotic and twenty-four hours later and she was back to her baseline.

But without that experience, without that knowledge, we might have assumed she had declined permanently. We might have assumed we were entering a new stage of the disease. We might have prepared ourselves for something irreversible when the problem was actually treatable.

Why UTIs Look So Different

In a healthy brain, a UTI causes:

- Burning
- Urgency
- Pain
- Fever
- Discomfort

But in a brain affected by Alzheimer's?

The part of the brain that interprets pain is damaged and weakened. The part that communicates symptoms is compromised.

So instead of saying: "It burns when I pee," or "I think I have an infection," your loved one will show you symptoms like:

- Sudden confusion
- Increased agitation
- Fearfulness
- Hallucinations
- Withdrawal
- Mood swings
- Refusal to eat
- Inability to walk
- Excessive sleepiness
- Physical collapse
- "Acting different" in a way you cannot explain

And those symptoms often look like: **rapid cognitive decline** instead of **infection.**

The medical term for this is *delirium*, and delirium in a dementia patient can look like the floor dropped out from under them. A good day can become a crisis in hours.

And without knowledge, families assume the worst:
- "When did she decline this much?"
- "Is this the next stage?"
- "Is this the beginning of the end?"
- "Did we miss something?"
- "Is this permanent?"

But very often, it's none of those things. It's a UTI.

Betty's Subtle (and Not-So-Subtle) Warning Signs
Every person shows UTIs differently, but my mother showed them in two ways.

1. A strong, unusual odor when she urinated
This was often the first sign. Not always, but often. An unmistakable change.

I cannot tell you how many times we said "Something's wrong. We think she has a UTI."

2. Sudden cognitive or physical decline

It was never slow. Never gradual. Never something we questioned for long.

It was abrupt, like someone flipped a switch.

One day she was herself, the next she was lost inside a deeper fog.

We learned to trust our instincts. We learned to act immediately. We learned to call the doctor first, and ask questions later.

Because once you've seen a UTI take down someone you love, once you've watched them disappear into confusion, you never again underestimate the power of a sudden change.

Why Caregivers Must Be Detectives

A person with dementia cannot report symptoms accurately. They cannot locate their pain. They cannot verbalize what feels wrong. They cannot describe why they feel off.

So you learn to become a detective, noticing the small things:

- Are they more confused today?
- Are they extra sleepy?
- Are they unusually agitated?
- Do they seem "not themselves"?
- Are they suddenly unsteady?
- Is there a smell in their urine?
- Are they refusing food unexpectedly?
- Are they scared for no reason?
- Did they mentally decline in hours, not weeks?

These questions become your new diagnostic tools.

You cannot rely on what they say. You must rely on what you see, smell, notice and what you feel.

Because caregivers develop an intuition, a deep knowing, that is more accurate than any symptom list.

Why UTIs Are So Common in Dementia

As dementia progresses, the risk of UTIs skyrockets for several reasons:

- Decreased mobility
- Difficulty emptying the bladder fully
- Incontinence
- Skin breakdown
- Dehydration
- Medication side effects
- Weakened immune response
- Reduced awareness of hygiene
- Increased use of adult diapers

Each of these creates the perfect environment for infection.

The more advanced the dementia, the more frequent the UTIs.

Sometimes it feels relentless. Sometimes it feels unfair. Sometimes it feels like the disease is attacking from every angle.

But knowledge gives you back a sense of control.

The Doctor Who Gave Us a Lifeline

Because Mom developed UTIs so often, and because the symptoms were dramatic, our doctor gave us something that truly changed our caregiving experience:

An antibiotic prescription we were allowed to keep on hand.

It was a game-changer.

No more waiting days for an appointment. No more emergency rooms. No more suffering while we begged someone to take her symptoms seriously.

We could start treatment immediately, with the doctor's guidance, and prevent a small infection from becoming a terrifying, disorienting crisis.

If your loved one has recurrent UTIs, talk to their doctor about this option. It may not be appropriate for everyone, but for us, it was essential.

How Many Crises We Avoided By Knowing The Signs

By the end of Mom's life, we had become so in tune with her behaviors that we could detect a UTI before it became severe.

- A slight shift in her eyes.
- A sudden difficulty standing.
- A moment of extreme fog.
- A strange odor.
- A change in her tone.
- A look of fear.

These were no longer mysteries, they were indicators.

We caught infections early. We treated them quickly. We prevented hospitalization. We prevented emotional trauma. We prevented physical decline.

And we prevented ourselves from assuming dementia progression when the problem was actually treatable.

The Raw Lesson Every Caregiver Must Learn

If you learn nothing else in this chapter, learn this:

In dementia caregiving, sudden changes are almost never "just dementia." Always check for a UTI.

It is one of the most common medical emergencies in dementia and one of the most easily misdiagnosed. Yet it is one of the most treatable.

You will save yourself fear.

You will save your loved one pain.

You will catch infections early.

You will prevent unnecessary suffering.

You will avoid misinterpreting decline.

And you will become more confident, more prepared, and more capable than you ever thought you could be.

LESSON 7:
RESPITE AND SUPPORT

"I wish someone had told me earlier that strength is not found in doing it alone, strength is found in knowing when you can't."

If there is a chapter that makes caregivers shift uncomfortably in their seats, it's this one.

Not because they don't understand it. But because they don't want to.

Caregivers, especially family caregivers, are some of the most selfless, devoted, quietly heroic people in the world. They give everything. They sacrifice themselves. They pour out every ounce of love, patience, and energy they have.

And they do it willingly.

But there's a truth every caregiver eventually collides with:

You cannot do this alone. And you are not meant to.

Asking for help is not weakness.

It is not failure.

It is not abandonment.

It is not neglect.

It is survival.

Caregiving for someone with Alzheimer's is not a one-person job. It is not a two-person job. It is a village-sized job. And even then, some days the village cracks.

But we didn't understand that at first. Or maybe we didn't want to.

Why We Thought We Could Do It Alone
My father is one of the most devoted husbands I've ever known. Loyal. Steady. Self-sacrificing. Old-school committed.

When Mom started declining, Dad and I handled everything ourselves. Together, but also separately.

Dad was on duty around the clock. I was on duty whenever I wasn't working or sleeping. We switched off without discussing it. We tag-teamed tasks without planning them. We built a routine without even realizing it.

For a while, it worked. At least... it seemed like it worked.

Dad rarely left the house for long. He refused overnight breaks. He felt responsible for her safety every minute.

And I was the bridge between them, supporting him, supporting her, supporting the household, supporting our sanity.

But slowly, day by day, we were draining ourselves dry. The signs were there. We just didn't want to see them.

The Breaking Point We Didn't Talk About
The hardest part of caring for Mom wasn't feeding her.

It wasn't the incontinence.

It wasn't the wandering, or the confusion, or the agitation.

It wasn't even the decline.

It was the **showers**.

Showers became the battlefield none of us wanted.

Mom resisted them with a strength that surprised us. She was terrified. She felt invaded. She felt overwhelmed. She felt confused.

We weren't just asking her to wash, we were asking her to surrender control in one of the most vulnerable moments a person can experience.

It broke Dad.

It broke me.

It broke her.

I remember one night in particular where Dad and I found each other upstairs, both of us crying.

We weren't crying because of the work. We weren't crying because of her resistance. We weren't crying because of the physical exhaustion.

We were crying because it hurt to watch someone we loved become afraid of the things she once did easily.

It broke Dad to see his wife afraid of him in that moment. It broke me to see him breaking.

But still, Dad resisted the idea of hiring help.

- "We can do it."
- "We don't need anyone."
- "She's my wife."
- "This is my job."
- "We're capable."

And we were.

But being capable isn't the same as being healthy.
Being capable isn't the same as being supported.
Being capable isn't the same as being okay.

The Day We Couldn't Do It Anymore
It was near the end of 2022 when I finally said it out
loud:

"Dad... we need help."

He resisted. He argued. He brushed it off.

Not because he didn't see the need, but because
admitting we needed help felt like admitting defeat.

It felt like failing her. Failing each other. Failing the
promise of a lifetime.

But we weren't failing. We were drowning.

The first step wasn't easy, but it was everything!

We hired part-time help, just two days a week, four
hours at a time. The caregiver would handle the
most difficult task of Mom's day: the shower.

And for those four hours, Dad and I would leave the house. We would breathe. We would go out to eat. We would go to the library and work on our laptops in silence. We would just... exist without the constant, unblinking vigilance.

And suddenly, the world felt survivable again.

Those small breaks were not luxuries. They were lifelines.

Without them, we might not have made it through the hardest days.

When Help Became Not Optional, But Essential
As the disease progressed, so did the help we needed.

Part-time support became full-time. Weekdays became weekends. Four hours became eight.

Eventually, our caregiver became one of the most important figures in our home.

She was gentle with Mom. Kind. Patient in ways we sometimes weren't capable of being.

She laughed with her. Held her hand. Listened to her. Talked to her. Let her dignity remain untouched even in the most vulnerable tasks.

And she gave Dad and me something we rarely felt:

Permission to rest.

Because here's the truth:

Caregiver burnout doesn't wait for permission. It takes your health whether you acknowledge it or not.

I have heard countless statistics about caregivers becoming ill, breaking down, or dying before the person they are caring for.

Some studies say as many as 40%. Even the lowest estimates are alarming.

Because caregiving, especially spousal caregiving, is physically draining, emotionally depleting, mentally exhausting, and spiritually heavy. I was terrified of dad dying before mom. She couldn't tolerate him being away in the bathroom for a few minutes, what if he were gone for good?

You cannot pour from an empty cup. But caregivers try anyway, until the cup cracks.

Why Asking for Help Is Not Failure

One of the most important shifts in my caregiving journey was accepting this truth:

I cannot save her alone. I can only love her well when I allow others to help me.

Respite is not abandonment. It is restoration.

Support is not weakness. It is wisdom.

Help is not an insult. It is a blessing.

And asking for help does not mean you love them any less. It means you love them enough to stay alive for the journey.

When you allow others to join your circle of care, you give yourself permission to be human.

To rest.

To breathe.

To recover.

To replenish what this disease drains from you every day.

And when you show up rested, your loved one feels it.

They trust you more. They relax more. They sense your calm. They lean into your steadiness.

Help doesn't make you a weaker caregiver. It makes you a better one.

Resources Caregivers Often Overlook
Many caregivers feel alone because they don't know where to turn.

But support exists, even if you don't have money, even if you don't have family nearby, even if you don't know where to start.

Some places to begin:
- County elder services
- Respite programs through local nonprofits
- The Alzheimer's Association
- Church volunteer groups
- Palliative care
- Hospice support when appropriate
- Adult day programs
- Friends or neighbors who genuinely want to help
- Family members who don't know what to do unless you ask

People often say, "Let me know if you need anything." But they don't know what you need. They aren't mind readers.

So tell them.

"Can you sit with her for two hours on Tuesday?"

"Can you pick up groceries this week?"

"Can you help me organize medication trays?"

People want to help. They just need guidance.

The Raw Lesson Every Caregiver Must Learn
Here is the truth this chapter wants to leave with you:

You cannot sacrifice your life to save theirs. You must preserve your health to protect theirs.

Rest is not optional. Support is not optional. Help is not optional.

Not if you want to make it through this disease with your heart intact.

There is no prize for doing it alone. There is no trophy for burning yourself out. There is no ribbon for never asking for help.

But there is a cost. And the cost is high.

Caregiving requires endurance. Endurance requires rest. Rest requires support.

It is not selfish to care for yourself. It is necessary.

And the greatest truth of all?

Your loved one would want you to survive this. And they would want you to live after they're gone.

You honor them when you take care of yourself.

You honor them when you let others help you.

You honor them when you preserve the parts of you that Alzheimer's tries to drain away.

This chapter is the seventh lesson because it is the one caregivers resist the longest. But it is the one that keeps you alive, physically, emotionally, and spiritually.

CONCLUSION:
LOVE OUTLASTS MEMORY

"The journey through dementia does not end where memory ends; it ends where love has given everything it can."

Dementia is a long journey, longer than any family ever expects. It begins quietly, whispers through the early years, then takes center stage in the later ones. It shifts identity, reshapes relationships, and requires a depth of love and patience that most of us never realized we possessed.

But as we've traveled through the seven stages together, one truth rises above all others:

Dementia can take memories, but it cannot take love.

It cannot touch the bond between parent and child, spouse and partner, grandparent and grandchild, caregiver and companion. It cannot erase the years you lived together or the stories you shared. It cannot silence laughter or eliminate the comfort of a familiar voice.

Dementia rearranges the landscape of a family's life, but it does not empty it of meaning. If anything, it deepens meaning.

It teaches:
- Patience that grows far beyond frustration
- Compassion that stretches beyond convenience
- Presence that replaces performance
- Love that becomes unconditional

Many caregivers describe dementia as the hardest thing they have ever lived through. Yet the same caregivers say they have never understood love more deeply.

Dementia becomes the teacher no one asked for, but its lessons shape hearts forever.

Caregiving in dementia is not about fixing. It's not about who remembers what. It's not about preventing decline. It's not about perfection.

It is about presence. It is about dignity. It is about humanity. It is about being there.

It is about choosing love when the world feels confusing, overwhelming, and unfair.

In the end, dementia doesn't define a person.

Their life does.

Their story does.

Their love does.

And your presence, your willingness to walk with them through every stage, becomes one of the greatest acts of love a human being can offer.

This conclusion is not the end of the story.

It is simply the beginning of understanding what it means to love someone through their final journey.

And here is the truth that every caregiver needs to hear:

You are doing better than you think you are.

You are stronger than you feel.

And you are not alone—not for one second of this journey.

When my mother took her last breath, and her hands finally loosened from the world, I realized something that will stay with me forever:

I thought I had been walking her home.

But the truth is, she was walking me home too.

She was shaping me into the son I needed to be, the caregiver I never imagined becoming, the man who could stand in the aftermath of loss and still recognize beauty, still choose compassion, still offer guidance to others.

Her journey didn't end when she died. It continues through me. It continues through this book. And now, in some small way, it continues through you.

As you care for your loved one, as you witness their changes, as you navigate the stages, as you shoulder the emotional weight of this disease, remember this:

You are honoring them in every moment.

You are loving them in every breath.

You are giving them dignity in every choice.

And **you are becoming someone braver than you ever knew you could be.**

CAREGIVER'S REFLECTION: WHAT THIS JOURNEY MEANT

*"Caregiving is not a role we choose…
it is a calling we grow into,
one quiet sacrifice at a time."*

Take a deep breath.

You have walked a long road.

Maybe you are still walking it.

Maybe you are somewhere in the middle, or maybe you have reached the end and are mourning the loss of someone who meant everything to you.

Wherever you are, this reflection is for you.

Caregiving is life changing.

Not just for the one receiving the care, but for the one giving it.

You learned things you never expected to learn…

How to bathe someone with dignity.

How to redirect gently instead of arguing.

How to calm fear with touch, not logic.

How to read emotions instead of words.

How to let go of frustration and cling to grace.

You discovered strength you didn't know you had...

The strength to wake up again.

The strength to face the same question fifty times.

The strength to cry in the shower, then return with a smile.

The strength to be patient with what feels unfair.

You experienced grief long before death arrived...

Grief for lost memories.

Grief for changed roles.

Grief for conversations that faded away.

Grief for the person slipping away in pieces.

This grief is real. It deserves space. It deserves compassion.

You also experienced beauty in unexpected places...

A smile on a hard day.

A moment of clarity.

A song that brought back memories.

A squeeze of the hand.

A peaceful sigh of recognition.

Dementia caregiving is not a burden, it is a calling.

Not everyone can do it.

But you did.

Or you are doing it now.

And it is shaping you into someone stronger, softer, wiser.

Take a moment to honor yourself.

Your love.

Your courage.

Your resilience.

Your willingness to show up, again and again.

This journey has transformed you.

And nothing, not dementia, not time, not loss, can take that transformation away.

How To Cope With Grief After Dementia

Grief enters the dementia journey long before the final breath.

This is called anticipatory grief: grieving someone who is still physically here but slowly slipping away.

And when they finally pass, the grief does not end. In many ways, it transforms.

Here is what caregivers often experience, and how to cope through each stage.

1. Grieving the Person Twice

Most caregivers grieve twice:

- During the disease, as pieces of the person change or fade
- After death, when the physical presence is gone

This double-loss is uniquely painful.

How to cope:

- Talk about your loved one often
- Allow yourself to feel whatever comes
- Write letters to them
- Share stories with family
- Keep something that brings comfort (a photo, a shirt, a keepsake)

Your grief is not only valid, it is sacred.

2. The "What If" Grief

Caregivers often replay decisions:

- "What if I had done this earlier?"
- "What if I missed something?"
- "What if I had been more patient?"
- "What if I failed them somehow?"

Let this truth wash over you:

You did the best you could with what you knew at the time. And **your best was enough.**

Dementia has no perfect choices. Only loving ones.

3. The Loss of Routine

Caregiving becomes a lifestyle.

When it ends, you lose not only the person, but the identity:

- The routines
- The responsibility
- The purpose
- The constant presence

This can leave caregivers feeling empty.

How to cope:
- Create new routines slowly
- Give yourself permission to rest
- Reconnect with hobbies and passions
- Seek community
- Volunteer or help others when ready

Healing takes time.

4. Guilt and Relief
- It is completely normal to feel:
- Relief that their suffering is over
- Relief that caregiving pressure has lifted
- Relief that they are at peace

And it is **normal to feel guilty** for feeling relief.

But the two emotions can live together.

Relief does not mean you loved them less.

Relief means you loved them deeply enough to know they deserved peace.

5. How to Heal
Healing is not linear.

Some days will be peaceful; others will feel heavy.

Here's what helps:

- Talk about your loved one: Stories keep them alive in our hearts.
- Join a grief or caregiver group: You need people who understand.
- Honor anniversaries gently: Light a candle. Say a prayer. Tell a story.
- Seek counseling if needed: Grief is not weakness. It is love with nowhere to go.

Remember what you did matters.

Caregiving is an act of love.

You changed their life.

And they changed yours.

RESOURCES & SUPPORT FOR CAREGIVERS

Here are the most trusted, helpful resources for dementia caregivers as well as ways you can help.

Alzheimer's Association
Website: alz.org

Offers 24/7 helplines, local support groups, educational materials, and resources for families.

Our Website
Website: ImBetty.com

Offers links to all our books, resources for caregivers, information on caregiver scholarships and links to helpful items when caring for someone with dementia.

Donate to the Alzheimer's Association
Please consider making a charitable donation to our Alzheimer's Association Fundraiser in honor of my mother, Betty, who inspired this book. A portion of every book sale goes to our fundraiser and to we have raised over $100,000. **You can find the link at our website, ImBetty.com.**

EPILOGUE:
THE LOVE THAT REMAINS

*"After the long goodbye is over,
what remains is not the disease,
but the love that carried you through it."*

When you reach the end of the dementia journey, you carry more than memories, you carry the weight of every moment you lived through, every decision you made, every tear you shed, and every act of love you offered on the days when you felt both strong and exhausted, hopeful and heartbroken.

You carry a story.

Not just the story of the one you cared for, but your own story as well, the story of a caregiver who showed up, day after day, even when the path felt impossible, even when your heart felt stretched thin, even when others could not understand the depth of what you were carrying.

This story, your story, is not defined by the disease.

It is defined by love.

Love in the early stages, when you noticed something wasn't quite right.

Love in the middle stages, when the questions repeated, when the nights were long, when the confusion grew.

Love in the later stages, when words faded, when recognition flickered, when your quiet presence mattered more than anything you could say.

Love in the final stage, when you held their hand, whispered your goodbyes, and released them with tenderness and grace.

This journey has asked much of you, but it has also shaped you.

Caregiving changes a person; it grows the heart in ways nothing else can.

You may feel different now.

You may feel older, softer, wiser.

You may feel broken in places, strong in others.

You may feel grief.

You may feel peace.

You may feel both.

But hear this truth: Nothing about the way you loved will ever be lost.

The person you cared for carried that love with them until their final breath.

And you carry the imprint of their life within your own.

Dementia may have rewritten parts of your story, but it did not erase the beauty of what was shared. Your journey together mattered. Every stage. Every step. Every moment.

Your love was seen.

Your love was felt.

Your love was enough.

ABOUT THE COVER PHOTO

*"The most powerful photographs are
not staged, they are simply
moments of love, caught in motion."*

In November of 2021, I rented a beach house in
Garden City, South Carolina for Thanksgiving week.
It was one of those rare windows in life when
everyone could be together. Mom and Dad were
there. My oldest brother, John, joined us. It was the
same trip when the now-famous "mirror video"
happened, the moment that unexpectedly changed
our lives and introduced Betty to the world.

The house was large, with extra bedrooms, so my
friend Tasha stayed with us for a few days as well. It
felt full, not just of people, but of warmth. Of time
we didn't yet realize was precious.

One afternoon, the weather shifted. The cool
November air gave way to sunshine and seventy-
degree warmth. It felt like a gift. The kind of day you
don't plan for but are grateful to receive.

The house sat directly on the beach. It came stocked with folding chairs, cornhole boards, and all the small things that make a beach day easy. So we carried everything down and settled into the sand. The ocean stretched wide and endless before us.

At that point, Mom was still fairly mobile. Walking wasn't impossible, just slower. But sand is unforgiving terrain, even for strong legs. For someone in the middle stages of Alzheimer's, it requires balance, coordination, and trust.

Dad and I looked at her and asked gently, "Do you want to walk down closer to the water?"

She smiled.

That smile said yes.

And in my heart, something whispered that this might be the last time she would walk in sand. The last time she would feel the pull of the tide up close. The last time she would stand at the edge of something vast and powerful and take it in with her own eyes.

So Dad and I each took a side.

We didn't rush. We didn't speak much. We just walked her forward, toward the horizon, toward the waves, toward the sound that has comforted generations before us.

Behind us, Tasha stayed back on the beach. At some point, she quietly lifted her phone and began snapping pictures. We weren't posing. We weren't trying to capture a moment. We were simply living it.

Later, when we saw the photos, we understood what she had captured.

Three figures walking toward the ocean.

Betty in the middle.

Supported on both sides.

Moving forward.

Facing the horizon.

You could not have staged something more symbolic if you tried.

The image carries layers that even we didn't fully grasp in that moment.

It speaks of **protection** — a mother once strong now gently supported by the son and husband who loved her.

It speaks of **transition** — the quiet crossing from independence to dependence, from strength to surrender.

It speaks of **journey** — not just that walk in the sand, but the eleven-year walk through Alzheimer's.

It speaks of **support** — two steady arms holding someone upright against shifting ground.

It speaks of **tender strength** — not dramatic, not heroic, just faithful.

And above all, it speaks of **walking someone home**.

When Mom later went viral, one of our followers saw that photo on Facebook and turned it into a canvas print. They sent it to us as a gift. We were overwhelmed. That canvas now hangs in my parents' bedroom, and it was displayed prominently at Betty's Celebration of Life. I wish I could remember who it was now, so I could send them a copy of this book as a thank you. Know that it touched us deeply.

Of all the images we have of her, smiling at the mirror, laughing in the kitchen, waving at the camera, **this one** feels different.

This one feels **eternal**.

It doesn't show Alzheimer's. It shows **love**.

It doesn't show decline. It shows **devotion**.

It doesn't show loss. It shows a family moving forward **together**, even when the ground beneath them was unsteady.

That day, we thought we were just walking to the water.

In truth, we were doing what we had been doing all along.

We were **walking her home**.

FINAL BLESSING & ENCOURAGEMENT

*"If you are walking this road now,
may you find strength for each day,
grace for each mistake, and the quiet
assurance that your love is enough."*

As you close this book, may these words settle gently on your heart.

May you find peace in knowing **you did everything you could**, not perfectly, not without weariness, but **with a love** that was deeper than the disease.

May you find rest after the long road you walked, rest for your mind, rest for your spirit, rest for your aching heart.

May you find comfort in the memories that remain, the laughter, the stories, the moments of clarity, the hands held tightly, the eyes that still sparkled with recognition.

May you let go of guilt, every caregiver carries it, but none of it belongs to you.

You loved. You gave. You showed up.

May you feel pride in the strength you found, the kind of strength that grows only in the heart of a caregiver, the kind of strength that comes from love.

May you carry forward the lessons this journey taught you, patience, compassion, tenderness, presence, resilience, humility, and the understanding that life's greatest treasures are often found in the smallest moments.

And finally...

May you remember that love does not end with memory.

Love outlasts forgetting.

Love outlasts decline.

Love outlasts death.

The love you gave, the love you received, the love you witnessed: it continues forward, living quietly and beautifully in you.

You were a blessing to the one you cared for.

And now, may you feel blessed in retur

FOLLOW US ON SOCIAL MEDIA

Follow our journey, memories and adventures on social media. We love hearing from followers and reading your comments and stories!

Email: Josh@ImBetty.com

@JoshuaPettit

@JoshPet

@JoshPet1975

@ImBettyPettit

@JoshPetNC